Magnetic Resonance Imaging in Deep Brain Stimulation

Alexandre Boutet • Andres M. Lozano
Editors

Magnetic Resonance Imaging in Deep Brain Stimulation

Springer

Editors
Alexandre Boutet
Joint Department of Medical Imaging
University of Toronto
Toronto, ON, Canada

Andres M. Lozano
Division of Neurosurgery
University Health Network and University
of Toronto
Toronto, ON, Canada

ISBN 978-3-031-16347-0 ISBN 978-3-031-16348-7 (eBook)
https://doi.org/10.1007/978-3-031-16348-7

This Springer imprint is published by the registered company Springer Nature Switzerland AG
The registered company address is: Gewerbestrasse 11, 6330 Cham, Switzerland

Preface

Several books have been written on DBS-related topics, primarily focusing on clinical and technical aspects of the treatment from neurological and neurosurgical perspectives. However, few of those books have focused on the role of neuroimaging, specifically MRI, in DBS surgery. With recent advances in neuroimaging technology and its increasingly prominent role, we felt that it would be timely for the DBS community to have an all-in-one resource summarizing the roles of MRI in DBS. We wanted to discuss the established as well as the innovative roles of MRI spanning the preoperative and postoperative care of these patients.

Over the past 25 years, the Toronto group has accumulated a large experience with DBS and has advanced several aspects of this field. Each chapter is written by local authors informed by our longstanding experience with DBS in Toronto. These were written in collaboration with international expert co-authors, who have ensured a thorough and global perspective on the topics covered.

We hope this book provides a succinct and clear summary of the various roles of MRI in DBS. It is our wish that the work herein sparks your interest so that you may further your knowledge of the topics using the references provided in each chapter. We believe that the roles of MRI in DBS will only grow over the next few years and will become increasingly central to most future clinical and research endeavours.

Toronto, ON, Canada Alexandre Boutet
Toronto, ON, Canada Andres M. Lozano

Contents

Deep Brain Stimulation and Magnetic Resonance Imaging: Introduction

1

Alexandre Boutet and Andres M. Lozano

In its broadest sense, functional neurosurgery includes the surgical treatment of pain, movement disorders, epilepsy, and psychiatric conditions. Fundamentally, the field is dedicated to treat pathological activity in circuits associated with a wide range of neurological conditions. Generally speaking, this can be achieved through stereotactic methods using lesioning or electrical stimulation of key brain structures. As a basic principle, the targeted structure represents a crucial hub within the circuit of interest: the motor circuit is targeted in Parkinson's disease, whereas structures implicated in mood regulation are targeted in psychiatric disorders and cognitive circuits in dementias and memory disorders [1].

Deep brain stimulation (DBS) has emerged as the dominant stereotactic functional neurosurgical procedure, in part due to its reversibility and also because it allows for the postoperative titration of electrical stimulation according to a patient's specific needs [2]. Following surgical insertion, an electrode placed into the desired brain target delivers controlled electrical stimulation, analogous in some ways to a cardiac pacemaker [3]. Most commonly employed in movement disorders such as Parkinson's disease, dystonia, and tremor, DBS is also being investigated for use in psychiatric and cognitive disorders, including depression and Alzheimer's disease [1, 2, 4]. It is estimated that more than 200,000 patients have undergone DBS surgery worldwide [4]. Imaging techniques, specifically magnetic resonance imaging (MRI), play central roles in the preoperative and postoperative aspects of DBS surgery.

A. Boutet (✉)
Joint Department of Medical Imaging, University of Toronto, Toronto, ON, Canada
e-mail: alexandre.boutet@mail.utoronto.ca

A. M. Lozano
Division of Neurosurgery, University Health Network and University of Toronto, Toronto, ON, Canada
e-mail: lozano@uhnresearch.ca

A. Boutet, A. M. Lozano (eds.), *Magnetic Resonance Imaging in Deep Brain Stimulation*, https://doi.org/10.1007/978-3-031-16348-7_1

During the preoperative period, MRI is critical for surgical planning, and the advent of novel MRI sequences now offer unparalleled visualization of DBS targets [3, 5]. Postoperatively, MRI can be used to assess electrode location and to model the local field of stimulation, while also permitting the investigation of clinical benefits and adverse events in terms of structural and functional anatomy. This can be done at the individual level, and more recently—thanks to advances in neuroimaging techniques—at the group level. Towards refining DBS therapy, group-level MRI-based probabilistic stimulation mapping is a powerful tool that leverages large amounts of historical data on targeting, programming, and clinical outcomes from past DBS interventions to be pooled and scrutinized [6, 7]. Furthermore, sequences such as functional MRI can now be acquired in DBS patients to investigate network engagement during active stimulation [8, 9]. This opens the door to a new field in neuromodulation research in which we can non-invasively probe the effects of brain stimulation in vivo. However, concerns over safety means that MRI in patients with DBS can only be performed under strict guidelines [10, 11]. Recent improvements in MRI and DBS safety knowledge have demonstrated that it is possible to acquire high resolution MRI in patients with DBS, thereby offering the potential to expand the possibilities of MRI and neuroimaging research in this population.

This book focuses on the established as well as the innovative roles of MRI in DBS. MRI and DBS are first introduced from an historical perspective and a review of the clinical aspects of DBS is performed. Then, the preoperative and postoperative applications of MRI in DBS are covered. The crucial aspect of MRI safety in these patients is also discussed. Finally, possible upcoming MRI applications for patients with DBS are discussed in a future directions chapter.

References

1. Lozano AM, Lipsman N. Probing and regulating dysfunctional circuits using deep brain stimulation. Neuron. 2013;77(3):406–24.
2. Lozano AM, Lipsman N, Bergman H, Brown P, Chabardes S, Chang JW, et al. Deep brain stimulation: current challenges and future directions. Nat Rev Neurol. 2019;15(3):148–60.
3. Krauss JK, Lipsman N, Aziz T, Boutet A, Brown P, Chang JW, et al. Technology of deep brain stimulation: current status and future directions. Nat Rev Neurol. 2021;17(2):75–87.
4. Vedam-Mai V, Deisseroth K, Giordano J, Lazaro-Munoz G, Chiong W, Suthana N, et al. Proceedings of the eighth annual deep brain stimulation think tank: advances in Optogenetics, ethical issues affecting DBS research, Neuromodulatory approaches for depression, adaptive Neurostimulation, and emerging DBS technologies. Front Hum Neurosci. 2021;15:644593.
5. Boutet A, Loh A, Chow CT, Taha A, Elias GJB, Neudorfer C, et al. A literature review of magnetic resonance imaging sequence advancements in visualizing functional neurosurgery targets. J Neurosurg. 2021:1–14. https://doi.org/10.3171/2020.8.JNS201125.
6. Elias GJB, Boutet A, Joel SE, Germann J, Gwun D, Neudorfer C, et al. Probabilistic mapping of deep brain stimulation: insights from 15 years of therapy. Ann Neurol. 2021;89(3):426–43.
7. Horn A, Reich M, Vorwerk J, Li N, Wenzel G, Fang Q, et al. Connectivity predicts deep brain stimulation outcome in Parkinson disease. Ann Neurol. 2017;82(1):67–78.
8. Boutet A, Madhavan R, Elias GJB, Joel SE, Gramer R, Ranjan M, et al. Predicting optimal deep brain stimulation parameters for Parkinson's disease using functional MRI and machine learning. Nat Commun. 2021;12(1):3043.

9. Elias GJB, Germann J, Boutet A, Loh A, Li B, Pancholi A, et al. 3 T MRI of rapid brain activity changes driven by subcallosal cingulate deep brain stimulation. Brain. 2022;145(6):2214–26.
10. Boutet A, Chow CT, Narang K, Elias GJB, Neudorfer C, Germann J, et al. Improving safety of MRI in patients with deep brain stimulation devices. Radiology. 2020;296(2):250–62.
11. Boutet A, Rashid T, Hancu I, Elias GJB, Gramer RM, Germann J, et al. Functional MRI safety and artifacts during deep brain stimulation: experience in 102 patients. Radiology. 2019;293(1):174–83.

A Historical Perspective on the Role of Imaging in Deep Brain Stimulation

2

Gavin J. B. Elias, Aazad Abbas, Aaron Loh, Jürgen Germann, and Michael L. Schwartz

Introduction

Deep brain stimulation (DBS) is a neurosurgical procedure in which metallic depth electrodes, connected by wires to an internalized battery, are implanted within the brain for the purpose of delivering ongoing trains of electrical pulses to specific neuroanatomical targets [1]. Implantation of DBS electrodes is performed in a minimally invasive, stereotactic fashion and relies on the use of brain imaging—typically acquired while the patient's head is fixed in a stereotactic frame—to select precise target coordinates prior to surgery. Electrode positioning is often adjusted intra-operatively based on electrophysiological recordings (microelectrode recording, MER) and test stimulation, and is usually confirmed intra-operatively and/or post-operatively with further imaging [2]. Once implanted, the electrodes are used to modulate dysfunctional brain activity on a chronic basis through both direct bioelectric effects on perielectrode cells and broader, network-level effects on oscillatory dynamics [3, 4] and cerebral metabolism and blood flow [5–8]. Unlike older functional neurosurgical therapies that achieve their effects by creating a physical and permanent lesion in the brain, DBS is notable for both its reversibility (i.e., stimulation can be turned on and off) and its titratability [9].

G. J. B. Elias · A. Abbas · A. Loh · J. Germann
Division of Neurosurgery, Department of Surgery, University Health Network and University of Toronto, Toronto, ON, Canada

Krembil Research Institute, University of Toronto, Toronto, ON, Canada

M. L. Schwartz (✉)
Division of Neurosurgery, Sunnybrook Health Sciences Centre, University of Toronto, Toronto, ON, Canada
e-mail: michael.schwartz@sunnybrook.ca

A. Boutet, A. M. Lozano (eds.), *Magnetic Resonance Imaging in Deep Brain Stimulation*, https://doi.org/10.1007/978-3-031-16348-7_2

Specifically, stimulation parameters such as amplitude/voltage, pulse width, and frequency can be selected and modified following implantation, allowing for therapy to be optimized for each patient on an individual basis.

While DBS in its modern incarnation emerged in the late 1990s, the technique grew out of older depth electrode work dating back to the 1970s [10–13]. These older studies tended to employ intracranial electrodes to deliver lower frequencies of stimulation (≤60 Hz), most commonly targeting structures such as periventricular/periaqueductal grey, sensory thalamus, and posterior limb of internal capsule for the treatment of refractory pain. It was discovered in 1987 that high-frequency (>100 Hz) stimulation mimicked the effect of lesional procedures (e.g., thalamotomy, pallidotomy, and subthalamotomy) [9], ushering in the widespread use of DBS for movement disorders such as Parkinson's disease (PD), essential tremor (ET), and dystonia in the 1990s [14–16]. Indeed, the efficacy and safety profile of DBS for movement disorders quickly established it as the neurosurgical procedure of choice for these conditions, largely supplanting the aforementioned ablative procedures [17–19]. In the decades since, DBS has seen continued, prevalent use for movement disorders and is also used clinically for refractory chronic pain and headache syndromes [20], epilepsy [21], Tourette syndrome [22], and obsessive-compulsive disorder [23]. In addition, DBS is presently under investigation for its utility in disorders such as treatment-resistant depression [24], anorexia nervosa [25], and Alzheimer's disease [26]. The wide variety of indications for DBS in part derives from the fact that stimulating electrodes may be inserted into different brain regions in order to modulate disease-relevant circuits and affect the desired symptoms [27]. The dorsolateral aspect of the subthalamic nucleus (STN)—a key hub in the brain's cortico-basal ganglia-thalamo-cortical motor circuit—is the primary target for PD [28], for instance, while the thalamic ventral intermediate nucleus (VIM) remains the preeminent target for ET [29].

It has long been understood that the therapeutic effects of DBS are mediated in the first instance through effects on the electrical dynamics of neurons and axons within a few millimeters of the implanted electrode [30]. Indeed, work in the early 2000s found electrode misplacement to be a frequent cause of poor clinical outcome following DBS surgery [31]. The importance of location to DBS outcome has been further emphasized in recent years by neuroimaging studies that demonstrated robust correlations between individual patient outcome and the location of implanted electrodes and/or volumes of tissue activated (VTA, the spatial extent of the direct bioelectric effect of stimulation) [32], and characterized "hotspots" of greater efficacy within existing targets [33]. For this reason, the accurate and precise positioning of electrodes within the target structure—a step that has always been inextricably bound to brain imaging—is paramount. In this chapter, we review the various imaging methods that have been used to facilitate DBS surgery over the decades, focusing on approaches taken to guide electrode placement for the treatment of major DBS indications. We discuss how these approaches have permitted either indirect or direct targeting techniques and touch upon recent imaging advances in the field of DBS.

Ventriculography

Ventriculography is the oldest imaging method that has been used to plan DBS surgeries [34]. This method involves the visualization of the cerebral ventricles and subarachnoid space with multiple plain radiographs (X-rays) following the drainage of CSF through an inserted spinal or intraventricular needle and its replacement with a substance (either air, gasses like oxygen or helium, or contrast media) that more clearly demarcates the ventricular borders. Having been injected with gas or contrast media, patients are rotated in varying positions over multiple hours, allowing for the injected substance to flow throughout the ventricular system and for intracranial targets to be fully mapped out. While ventriculography provides precise and undistorted images of the cerebral ventricles and constituted an improvement on preexisting skull radiography, it was historically associated with adverse outcomes such as patient discomfort and headaches, contrast reactions, and the risk of CSF leakage and hemorrhage [35–37]. A key feature of ventriculography-based stereotactic targeting is that it is by necessity *indirect*; DBS target structures such as STN cannot be visualized on the X-ray images themselves but must instead be localized based on contextual spatial relationships with visible landmarks (i.e., the anterior commissure (AC), posterior commissure (PC), and other structures bordering the third ventricle) (Fig. 2.1). In practice, this has involved the application of stereotactic diagrams [38–40] or atlases [41, 42] that indicate the likely location of target structures on the basis of prior anatomical and/or clinical studies, and which must be fitted or deformed to the coordinate space defined by the visualized periventricular landmarks [43]. Given that indirect targeting does not take into account individual variability in location, size, or shape of the target structure [44], intraoperative adjustment or "secondary targeting" by way of test stimulation and MER has classically been essential for accurate electrode placement.

Ventriculography was first described by American neurosurgeon Walter Dandy in 1919 [34] and was adopted for initial use in stereotactic procedures (using iodine rather than air) by Jean Talairach in the 1940s and 1950s [45]. Talairach also identified AC and PC as stereotactic reference points for a brain coordinate system at this time, based on the fact that they were clearly identifiable on ventriculography images; indeed, these structures have remained the gold standard landmarks for indirect neurosurgical targeting using other imaging modalities to the present day [46]. The German neurologists Hans Orthner and Fritz Roeder subsequently introduced stereotactic air ventriculography in the 1950s, seeking to avoid the potentially hazardous effects associated with iodine contrast injection (e.g. iodine hypersensitivity, epileptic seizures, and aqueductal stenosis). They also introduced the practice of mounting the stereotactic frame and performing the ventriculography procedure under general anesthesia to improve patient comfort, as well as the use of a "one stage" ventriculography (as opposed to two stage) approach on the day of surgery itself. Avoiding inaccuracies associated with readjusting the frame to the central ray and realigning the X-rays, the one stage procedure led to enhanced targeting accuracy and improved outcomes and soon became the preferred approach [47–50]. Further advancements came in the 1960s, when the Canadian team of Ronald

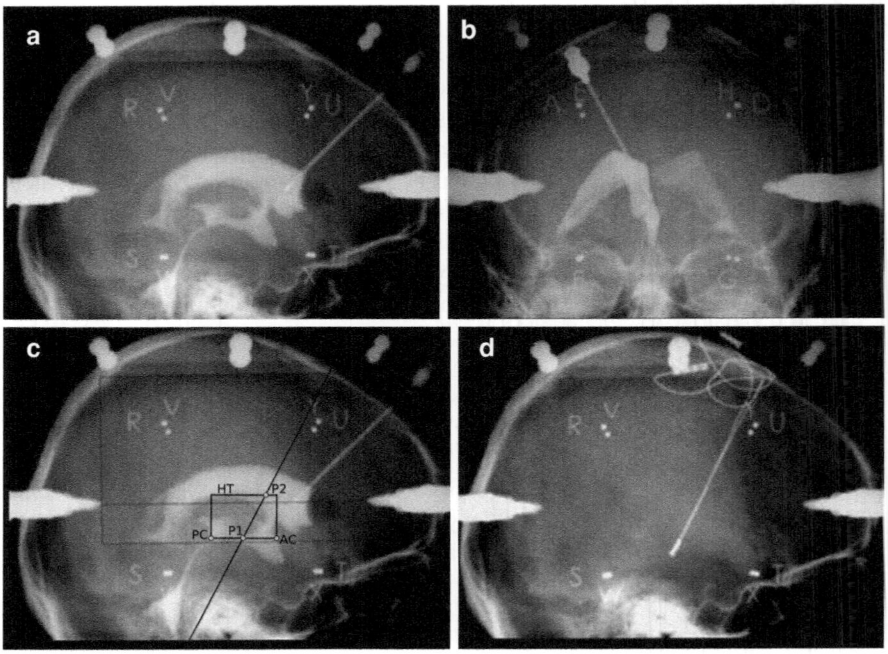

Fig. 2.1 DBS targeting using pre-operative ventriculography. (**a**) Representative lateral and (**b**) frontal views of stereotactic pre-operative contrast ventriculograms, permitting visualization of the ventricles and periventricular landmarks. A cannula can be seen in the frontal horn of the right lateral ventricle. (**c**) A popular method of indirect targeting, indicated by superimposed lines and circles, was used to target the subthalamic nucleus (STN) [60]. First, the anterior commissure (AC), posterior commissure (PC), and height (i.e., top) of the thalamus (HT, as indicated by the floor of the lateral ventricle) were identified. Subsequently, auxiliary points P1 and P2 were determined at the midcommissural point and five/sixth of the distance from PC to AC on the HT line, respectively. The STN target point was defined in the y and z planes as the intersection point of the line passing through P1 and P2 and the floor of the third ventricle, while the x coordinate of this point was typically given as 12 mm lateral to the midplane of the third ventricle (as visualized on the frontal ventriculogram). (**d**) A lateral post-operative X-ray shows DBS electrodes implanted using this targeting method. Panels A and B are reprinted with permission from Benabid AL, Mitrofanis J, Chabardes S, et al. Subthalamic Nucleus Stimulation for Parkinson's Disease. In: Lozano AM, Gildenberg PL, Tasker RR, editors. Textbook of Stereotactic and Functional Neurosurgery [Internet]. Berlin, Heidelberg: Springer; 2009 [cited 2022 Mar 8]. p. 1603–30. Panel C is adapted with minor edits from the same source. Panel D is reprinted with permission from Benabid AL, Chabardes S, Mitrofanis J, et al. Deep brain stimulation of the subthalamic nucleus for the treatment of Parkinson's disease. Lancet Neurol. 2009;8 (1):67–81

Tasker, Leslie Organ, and Peter Hawrylyshyn used ventriculography in conjunction with intra-operative stimulation to meticulously map somatosensory responses in the thalamus and midbrain. This allowed them to refine the dimensions of the popular Schaltenbrand and Bailey atlas and contributed to improved accuracy in indirect stereotactic targeting going forward [51, 52].

Prior to the widespread adoption of CT and MRI techniques in the 1970s and 1980s, ventriculography was the only viable means of precisely visualizing intracranial features. As such, it was performed extensively to guide a variety of stereotactic neurosurgical procedures, including early depth electrode work in patients with chronic pain [53] and other conditions [13]. Even as modern high-frequency DBS gathered steam in the 1990s, however, ventriculography remained in use. While the risks associated with the invasive procedure were increasingly highlighted in the context of non-invasive radiological alternatives [54], many functional neurosurgeons considered it the "gold standard" into the early 2000s [9]. This enduring preference in the face of more modern modalities was rooted not only in the technique's decades of proven use as a stereotactic tool, but also in the understanding that ventriculography avoided major image distortions (other than magnification caused by the conic projection of X-ray images onto photographic film) [55]. As a result of these sentiments, an era of overlap ensued in which ventriculography was often combined with CT or MRI for targeting purposes [56]. A 2008 systematic review of targeting methods revealed that, of the almost 500 STN-DBS patients reported on during the 1990s and early 2000s, over one-third underwent surgeries guided by ventriculography in combination with another imaging modality [57].

Modern Neuroimaging Techniques: Magnetic Resonance Imaging and Computed Tomography

As previously mentioned, the 1970s and 1980s saw the introduction of two novel techniques that revolutionized neuroimaging. Computed tomography (CT) imaging, a technique that uses tomographic reconstruction and a rotating array of X-ray generators and detectors to generate a series of cross-sectional images through a given object, was first introduced as a clinical neuroimaging tool in the early 1970s after its invention by Sir Godfrey Hounsfield [58]. Approximately a decade later, magnetic resonance imaging (MRI), a wholly separate, non-radiation-based technique that employs magnetic fields and radiofrequency pulses to detect a variety of (proton spin-related) properties of scanned tissues, emerged as a radiological tool [59]. Both methods boasted clear advantages over ventriculography in that they were non-invasive (and thus less dangerous for patients), generated three-dimensional images, and permitted unprecedented visualization of parenchymal structures [59]. Nonetheless, both CT and MRI were subjected to initial scrutiny and numerous head-to-head comparisons with ventriculography [54, 60–63] before either became accepted as reliable modes of imaging for guiding stereotactic surgery. As mentioned earlier, a period of overlap ensued during the 1990s and 2000s in which various groups planned DBS surgeries using either CT or MRI alone, CT and MRI in combination, or either method in combination with ventriculography [57]. Gradually, most centers adopted MRI—either alone or in conjunction with CT—as their pre-operative imaging method of choice. To this day, some groups elect to plan DBS surgeries on the basis of stereotactic MRI alone, while others acquire MRI at an earlier time and fuse (coregister) this image to a stereotactic CT scan, often using proprietary planning software [64]. The main justification for combining the two techniques has been to avoid the risk of susceptibility artifacts produced on MRI by the metallic stereotactic head frame, which some have argued distort the image and negatively impact targeting accuracy [65]. While there is research to suggest that solely MRI-guided targeting does not impair the accuracy of electrode implantation [65] and—in the case of 1.5 T MRI—results in similar electrode coordinates to MRI/CT fusion-based targeting [66], MRI/CT fusion remains the preferred method for many DBS surgeons, especially when 3 T MRI (which may be more prone to susceptibility-related distortion) is employed.

Overall, several factors appeared to drive the trend towards increased reliance on pre-operative MRI targeting throughout the 1990s and 2000s. For one, there was growing recognition that neuroanatomical landmarks for indirect targeting—visible on both CT and MRI, as they were on ventriculography—could be visualized with greater detail on MRI. Indeed, MRI was noted in the early 2000s to permit not only good visualization of AC and PC, which remained the leading anatomical fiducials for DBS implantation [46], but also the use of new, STN-adjacent landmarks like the red nucleus [67]. Another unique advantage of MRI was the ability to visualize DBS targets such as STN and GPi directly for the first time on pre-operative imaging (i.e., *direct* targeting) [2]. This was possible in large part due to the potential to customize MRI sequences to emphasize specific tissue contrasts. The early 2000s saw particular interest in the use of T2-weighted MRI to directly visualize the STN as a hypointense region located lateral to the red nucleus and dorsolateral to the substantia nigra. Several papers established T2-weighted MRI as sufficient guidance for consistent and accurate electrode placements, although they also noted the sequence's inability to reliably visualize the posterior aspect of STN (due to its decreased iron content) [68–70]. The safety and efficacy of T2-weighted MRI was also demonstrated at this time through post-operative follow-up of improvement of motor scores and activities of daily living [71]. Inversion recovery (IR) sequences also received extensive attention with regard to STN visualization in the early 2000s; several studies showed these to be similarly useful to T2-weighted images for identifying STN borders, with potential synergistic applications [72, 73]. One particular IR sequence—the FGATIR (fast gray matter acquisition T1 IR), developed in 2009—was notable for its applications to not only STN but also other DBS targets such as GPi, external globus pallidus, and thalamus [74]. Additional sequences of interest such as T2* [75] and susceptibility-weighted imaging (SWI) [76] were also explored in the 2000s due to their increased sensitivity to local STN iron deposits [70], with reported improvements in STN visualization and delimitation. Overall, the growing adoption of direct MRI imaging in DBS can be traced in the timeline of studies comparing indirect and direct MRI targeting throughout the 2000s; while earlier papers tended to favor indirect methods in terms of accuracy and precision [60, 77, 78], this trend reversed course in subsequent years [79–82]. Mounting evidence in this period also corroborated both the existence of clinically meaningful interindividual variability in the size and position of common DBS targets and the ability for these structures to be directly targeted using MRI [83–85]. Notably, the adoption of higher field strength MRI—particularly the clinical uptake of 3 T MRI following FDA approval in 2000 [86]—has also served to bolster the direct targeting approach due to its enhanced signal-to-noise ratio compared to 1.5 T MRI [87].

Recent Advances in DBS Neuroimaging

Today, MRI alone or combined MRI/CT continues to be the modality of choice for pre-operative planning of DBS surgeries. There is a great deal of ongoing research focused on further optimizing and expanding the use of MRI as a targeting tool. These include the development of new MRI sequences such as quantitative-susceptibility mapping, the application of ultra-high field DBS (i.e., ≥7 T), the adoption of structural (diffusion-weighted MRI) and functional (functional MRI) network-based MRI targeting, and the use of insights from large-scale DBS analyses incorporating probabilistic mapping and normative connectomic techniques [33, 88, 89]. The continued development of new MRI sequences and use of ultra-high field DBS have contributed to improvements in direct targeting and opened the door to direct visualization of thalamic nuclei such as VIM [90]. The mounting interest in functional and particularly diffusion-weighted MRI—popularized by researchers such as Volker Coenen in the early 2010s [91]—is noteworthy given that these modalities shift the focus away from discrete target nuclei and towards a broader, circuit-based conception of neurological conditions [92]. From a practical perspective, they have opened the door to visualizing previously "unseen" neuroanatomical entities; diffusion-weighted MRI tractography, for instance, has been used to triangulate and target specific white matter bundles for treatment of refractory depression [93] and obsessive-compulsive disorder [94] and to directly stimulate the dentato-rubro-thalamic tract for control of tremor [91, 95]. Probabilistic stimulation mapping—an approach in which clinical outcome and electrode/VTA location data from prior cases are aggregated and probed for spatial trends in a common imaging space using voxel-wise analysis techniques—has also blossomed in recent years following incipient work in the early 2010s [96], with various groups conducting large-scale studies to identify empirical "hotspots" of efficacy for stimulation that could be used to guide and refine future targeting [33, 97, 98]. Finally, building on seminal work by Andreas Horn in 2017 [99], a growing number of researchers have turned to "big data" analyses of DBS network engagement using diffusion-weighted and functional MRI data from large numbers of healthy individuals ("normative connectomes"). This approach has allowed connectivity-based research questions to be addressed in DBS populations that lack native connectivity imaging, with important implications for understanding this therapy's mechanism of action and for further optimizing its delivery [89]. Subsequent chapters in this book will discuss these various ongoing research initiatives in greater depth.

References

1. Lozano AM, Eltahawy H. How does DBS work? Suppl Clin Neurophysiol. 2004;57:733–6.
2. Brunenberg EJL, Platel B, Hofman PAM, ter Haar Romeny BM, Visser-Vandewalle V. Magnetic resonance imaging techniques for visualization of the subthalamic nucleus: a review. JNS. 2011;115(5):971–84.
3. McIntyre CC, Grill WM, Sherman DL, Thakor NV. Cellular effects of deep brain stimulation: model-based analysis of activation and inhibition. J Neurophysiol. 2004;91(4):1457–69
4. Birdno MJ, Grill WM. Mechanisms of deep brain stimulation in movement disorders as revealed by changes in stimulus frequency. Neurotherapeutics. 2008;5(1):14–25.
5. Hilker R, Voges J, Weber T, Kracht LW, Roggendorf J, Baudrexel S, et al. STN-DBS activates the target area in Parkinson disease: an FDG-PET study. Neurology. 2008;71(10):708–13.
6. Elias GJB, Germann J, Boutet A, Pancholi A, Beyn ME, Bhatia K, et al. Structuro-functional surrogates of response to subcallosal cingulate deep brain stimulation for depression. Brain [Internet]. 2021 [cited 2021 Aug 28];(awab284). Available from: https://doi.org/10.1093/brain/awab284.
7. Hershey T, Revilla FJ, Wernle AR, McGee-Minnich L, Antenor JV, Videen TO, et al. Cortical and subcortical blood flow effects of subthalamic nucleus stimulation in PD. Neurology. 2003;61(6):816–21.
8. Laxton AW, Tang-Wai DF, McAndrews MP, Zumsteg D, Wennberg R, Keren R, et al. A phase I trial of deep brain stimulation of memory circuits in Alzheimer's disease. Ann Neurol. 2010;68(4):521–34.
9. Benabid AL. Deep brain stimulation for Parkinson's disease. Curr Opin Neurobiol. 2003;13(6):696–706.
10. Hosobuchi Y, Adams JE, Rutkin B. Chronic thalamic stimulation for the control of facial anesthesia dolorosa. Arch Neurol. 1973;29(3):158–61.
11. Adams JE, Hosobuchi Y, Fields HL. Stimulation gof internal capsule for relief of chronic pain. J Neurosur. 1974;41:740–4.
12. Richardson DE, Akil H. Pain reduction by electrical brain stimulation in man. Part 1: acute administration in periaqueductal and periventricular sites. J Neurosurg. 1977;47(2):178–83.
13. Cooper IS, Upton AR, Amin I. Reversibility of chronic neurologic deficits. Some effects of electrical stimulation of the thalamus and internal capsule in man. Appl Neurophysiol. 1980;43(3–5):244–58.
14. Benabid AL, Pollack P, Gervason C, Hoffman D, Gao DM, Hommel M, et al. Long term suppression of tremor by chronic stimulation of the ventral intermediate thalamic nucleus. Lancet. 1991;337:403–6.
15. Limousin P, Pollak P, Benazzouz A, Hoffmann D, Le Bas JF, Broussolle E, et al. Effect of parkinsonian signs and symptoms of bilateral subthalamic nucleus stimulation. Lancet. 1995;345(8942):91–5.
16. Siegfried J, Lippitz B. Bilateral chronic electrostimulation of ventroposterolateral pallidum: a new therapeutic approach for alleviating all parkinsonian symptoms. Neurosurgery. 1994;35(6):1126–9. discussion 1129–1130.
17. Sandoe C, Krishna V, Basha D, Sammartino F, Tatsch J, Picillo M, et al. Predictors of deep brain stimulation outcome in tremor patients. Brain Stimul. 2018;11(3):592–9.
18. Moro E, Lozano AM, Pollak P, Agid Y, Rehncrona S, Volkmann J, et al. Long-term results of a multicenter study on subthalamic and pallidal stimulation in Parkinson's disease. Mov Disord. 2010;25(5):578–86.
19. Meoni S, Fraix V, Castrioto A, Benabid AL, Seigneuret E, Vercueil L, et al. Pallidal deep brain stimulation for dystonia: a long term study. J Neurol Neurosurg Psychiatry. 2017;88(11):960–7.
20. Levy RM, Lamb S, Adams JE. Treatment of chronic pain by deep brain stimulation: long term follow-up and review of the literature. Neurosurgery. 1987;21:885–93.
21. Andrade DM, Zumsteg D, Hamani C, Hodaie M, Sarkissian S, Lozano AM, et al. Long-term follow-up of patients with thalamic deep brain stimulation for epilepsy. Neurology. 2006;66(10):1571–3.

22. Ackermans L, Temel Y, Visser-Vandewalle V. Deep brain stimulation in Tourette's syndrome. Neurotherapeutics. 2008;5(2):339–44.
23. Roh D, Chang WS, Chang JW, Kim CH. Long-term follow-up of deep brain stimulation for refractory obsessive-compulsive disorder. Psychiatry Res. 2012;200(2–3):1067–70.
24. Kennedy SH, Giacobbe P, Rizvi SJ, Placenza FM, Nishikawa Y, Mayberg HS, et al. Deep brain stimulation for treatment-resistant depression: follow-up after 3 to 6 years. Am J Psychiatry. 2011;168(5):502–10.
25. De Vloo P, Lam E, Elias GJ, Boutet A, Sutandar K, Giacobbe P, et al. Long-term follow-up of deep brain stimulation for anorexia nervosa. J Neurol Neurosurg Psychiatry [Internet]. 2021; Mar 8 [cited 2021 Mar 10]; Available from: https://jnnp.bmj.com/content/early/2021/03/08/jnnp-2020-325711
26. Lozano AM, Fosdick L, Chakravarty MM, Leoutsakos JM, Munro C, Oh E, et al. A phase II study of fornix deep brain stimulation in mild Alzheimer's disease. J Alzheimers Dis. 2016;54(2):777–87.
27. Lozano A, Lipsman N. Probing and regulating dysfunctional circuits using deep brain stimulation. Neuron. 2013;77(3):406–24.
28. Okun MS. Deep-brain stimulation for Parkinson's disease. N Engl J Med. 2012;367(16):1529–38.
29. Baizabal-Carvallo JF, Kagnoff MN, Jimenez-Shahed J, Fekete R, Jankovic J. The safety and efficacy of thalamic deep brain stimulation in essential tremor: 10 years and beyond. J Neurol Neurosurg Psychiatry. 2014;85(5):567–72.
30. Jakobs M, Fomenko A, Lozano AM, Kiening KL. Cellular, molecular, and clinical mechanisms of action of deep brain stimulation—a systematic review on established indications and outlook on future developments. EMBO Mol Med. 2019;11(4):e9575.
31. Okun MS, Tagliati M, Pourfar M, Fernandez HH, Rodriguez RL, Alterman RL, et al. Management of referred deep brain stimulation failures: a retrospective analysis from 2 movement disorders centers. Arch Neurol. 2005 Aug;62(8):1250–5.
32. Yousif N, Purswani N, Bayford R, Nandi D, Bain P, Liu X. Evaluating the impact of the deep brain stimulation induced electric field on subthalamic neurons: a computational modelling study. J Neurosci Methods. 2010;188(1):105–12.
33. Elias GJB, Boutet A, Joel SE, Germann J, Gwun D, Neudorfer C, et al. Probabilistic mapping of deep brain stimulation: insights from 15 years of therapy. Ann Neurol. 2021;89(3):426–43.
34. Hamel W, Köppen JA, Hariz M, Krack P, Moll CKE. The pioneering and unknown stereotactic approach of Roeder and Orthner from Göttingen. Part I. surgical technique for tailoring individualized stereotactic lesions. Stereotact Funct Neurosurg. 2016;94(4):240–53.
35. Cheshire WP, Ehle AL. Hemiparkinsonism as a complication of an Ommaya reservoir: case report. J Neurosurg. 1990;73(5):774–6.
36. Marks PV, Wild AM, Gleave JRW. Long-term abolition of parkinsonian tremor following attempted ventriculography. Br J Neurosurg. 1991;5(5):505–8.
37. Hoeffner EG, Mukherji SK, Srinivasan A, Quint DJ. Neuroradiology Back to the future: brain imaging. AJNR Am J Neuroradiol. 2012;33(1):5–11.
38. Benabid AL, Koudsie A, Benazzouz A, Le Bas JF, Pollak P. Imaging of subthalamic nucleus and ventralis intermedius of the thalamus. Mov Disord. 2002;17(Suppl 3):S123–9.
39. Benabid AL, Mitrofanis J, Chabardes S, Seigneuret E, Torres N, Piallat B, et al. Subthalamic nucleus stimulation for Parkinson's disease. In: Lozano AM, Gildenberg PL, Tasker RR, editors. Textbook of stereotactic and Functional Neurosurgery [Internet]. Berlin, Heidelberg: Springer; 2009 [cited 2022 Mar 8]. p. 1603–30. Available from: https://doi.org/10.1007/978-3-540-69960-6_96.
40. Benabid AL, Chabardes S, Mitrofanis J, Pollak P. Deep brain stimulation of the subthalamic nucleus for the treatment of Parkinson's disease. Lancet Neurol. 2009 Jan;8(1):67–81.
41. Schaltenbrand G, Bailey P. Einführung in die stereotaktischen Operationen, mit einem atlas des menschlichen Gehirns. Introduction to stereotaxis, with an atlas of the human brain. Stuttgart: Thieme; 1959.
42. Schaltenbrand G, Wahren W, Hassler RG. Atlas for stereotaxy of the human brain: with an accompanying guide. Architectonic organization of the thalamic nuclei by Rolf Hassler 2, rev. and enlarged ed. Stuttgart: Thieme; 1977.

43. Caire F, Ouchchane L, Coste J, Gabrillargues J, Derost P, Ulla M, et al. Subthalamic nucleus location: relationships between stereotactic AC-PC-based diagrams and MRI anatomy-based contours. Stereotact Funct Neurosurg. 2009;87(6):337–47.
44. Hamid NA. Targeting the subthalamic nucleus for deep brain stimulation: technical approach and fusion of pre- and postoperative MR images to define accuracy of lead placement. J Neurol Neurosurg Psychiatry. 2005;76(3):409–14.
45. Mazoyer B. Jean Talairach (1911–2007): a life in stereotaxy. Hum Brain Mapp. 2008;29(2):250–2.
46. Starr PA, Christine CW, Theodosopoulos PV, Lindsey N, Byrd D, Mosley A, et al. Implantation of deep brain stimulators into the subthalamic nucleus: technical approach and magnetic resonance imaging-verified lead locations. J Neurosurg. 2002;97(2):370–87.
47. Orthner H, Roeder F. Experiences with stereotactic surgery. IV. Onthe long-term effect of bilateral pallidotomy in Parkinson's syndrome. Acta Neurochir. 1962;10:572–629.
48. Schmidt K, Dieckmann G, Prager J. On displacements of intracranial structures dependent on location by pneumoencephalography and during stereotactic brain surgery. A contribution to the technic of stereotactic brain surgery. Acta Neurochir. 1965;13(1):11–26.
49. Horwitz NH. Positive contrast ventriculography; a critical evaluation. J Neurosurg. 1956;13(4):300–11.
50. Redfern RM. History of stereotactic surgery for Parkinson's disease. Br J Neurosurg. 1989;3(3):271–304.
51. Hawrylyshyn PA, Tasker RR, Organ LW. Third ventricular width and the thalamocapsular border. Appl Neurophysiol. 1976/1977;39(1):34–42.
52. Tasker RR, Organ LW, Hawrylyshyn PA. The thalamus and midbrain of man: a physiological atlas using electrical stimulation. Springfield, Ill: C.C. Thomas; 1982. 505p. (American lecture series).
53. Fields HL, Adams JE. Pain after cortical injury relieved by electrical stimulation of the internal capsule. Brain. 1974;97(1):169–78.
54. Alterman RL, Kall BA, Cohen H, Kelly PJ. Stereotactic ventrolateral thalamotomy: is ventriculography necessary? Neurosurgery. 1995;37(4):717–21. discussion 721–722.
55. Benabid AL, Benazzouz A, Gao D, Hoffmann D, Limousin P, Koudsie A, et al. Chronic Electrical Stimulation of the Ventralis Intermedius Nucleus of the Thalamus and of Other Nuclei as a Treatment for Parkinson's Disease: Techniques in Neurosurgery 1999 5(1):5–30.
56. Limousin P, Krack P, Pollak P, Benazzouz A, Ardouin C, Hoffmann D, et al. Electrical stimulation of the subthalamic nucleus in advanced Parkinson's disease. N Engl J Med. 1998;339(16):1105–11.
57. Temel Y, Prinsenberg T, Visser-Vandewalle V. Imaging of the subthalamic nucleus for deep brain stimulation: a systematic review. Neuromodulation. 2008;11(1):8–12.
58. Richmond C. Sir Godfrey Hounsfield. BMJ. 2004;329(7467):687.1.
59. Kim PE, Zee CS. Imaging of the cerebrum. Neurosurgery. 2007;61(1 Suppl):123–46. discussion 146.
60. Breit S, LeBas JF, Koudsie A, Schulz J, Benazzouz A, Pollak P, et al. Pretargeting for the implantation of stimulation electrodes into the subthalamic nucleus: a comparative study of magnetic resonance imaging and ventriculography. Oper Neurosurgery. 2006;58(suppl_1) ONS-83–ONS-95.
61. Hariz MI, Bergenheim AT. A comparative study on ventriculographic and computerized tomography-guided determinations of brain targets in functional stereotaxis. J Neurosurg. 1990;73(4):565–71.
62. Hariz MI, Bergenheim AT, Fodstad H. Air-ventriculography provokes an anterior displacement of the third ventricle during functional stereotactic procedures. Acta Neurochir. 1993;123(3–4):147–52.
63. Schuurman PR, de Bie RM, Majoie CB, Speelman JD, Bosch DA. A prospective comparison between three-dimensional magnetic resonance imaging and ventriculography for target-coordinate determination in frame-based functional stereotactic neurosurgery. J Neurosurg. 1999;91(6):911–4.

64. Burke JF, Tanzillo D, Starr PA, Lim DA, Larson PS. CT and MRI image fusion error: an analysis of co-registration error using commercially available deep brain stimulation surgical planning software. Stereotact Funct Neurosurg. 2021;99(3):196–202.
65. Simon SL, Douglas P, Baltuch GH, Jaggi JL. Error analysis of MRI and leksell stereotactic frame target localization in deep brain stimulation surgery. Stereotact Funct Neurosurg. 2005;83(1):1–5.
66. Pezeshkian P, DeSalles AAF, Gorgulho A, Behnke E, McArthur D, Bari A. Accuracy of frame-based stereotactic magnetic resonance imaging vs frame-based stereotactic head computed tomography fused with recent magnetic resonance imaging for postimplantation deep brain stimulator lead localization. Neurosurgery. 2011;69(6):1299–306.
67. Aziz TZ, Nandi D, Parkin S, Liu X, Giladi N, Bain P, et al. Targeting the subthalamic nucleus. Stereotact Funct Neurosurg. 2001;77(1–4):87–90.
68. Starr PA, Vitek JL, DeLong M, Bakay RA. Magnetic resonance imaging-based stereotactic localization of the globus pallidus and subthalamic nucleus. Neurosurgery. 1999;44(2):303–13. discussion 313–314.
69. Egidi M, Rampini P, Locatelli M, Farabola M, Priori A, Pesenti A, et al. Visualisation of the subthalamic nucleus: a multiple sequential image fusion (MuSIF) technique for direct stereotaxic localisation and postoperative control. Neurol Sci. 2002;23(0)):s71–2.
70. Dormont D, Ricciardi KG, Tandé D, Parain K, Menuel C, Galanaud D, et al. Is the subthalamic nucleus hypointense on T2-weighted images? A correlation study using MR imaging and stereotactic atlas data. AJNR Am J Neuroradiol. 2004;25(9):1516–23.
71. Patel NK, Plaha P, O'Sullivan K, McCarter R, Heywood P, Gill SS. MRI directed bilateral stimulation of the subthalamic nucleus in patients with Parkinson's disease. J Neurol Neurosurg Psychiatry. 2003;74(12):1631–7.
72. Ishimori T, Nakano S, Mori Y, Seo R, Togami T, Masada T, et al. Preoperative identification of subthalamic nucleus for deep brain stimulation using three-dimensional phase sensitive inversion recovery technique. Magn Reson Med Sci. 2007;6(4):225–9.
73. Kitajima M, Korogi Y, Kakeda S, Moriya J, Ohnari N, Sato T, et al. Human subthalamic nucleus: evaluation with high-resolution MR imaging at 3.0 T. Neuroradiology. 2008;50(8):675–81.
74. Sudhyadhom A, Haq IU, Foote KD, Okun MS, Bova FJ. A high resolution and high contrast MRI for differentiation of subcortical structures for DBS targeting: the fast gray matter acquisition T1 inversion recovery (FGATIR). NeuroImage. 2009;47(Suppl 2):T44–52.
75. Elolf E, Bockermann V, Gringel T, Knauth M, Dechent P, Helms G. Improved visibility of the subthalamic nucleus on high-resolution stereotactic MR imaging by added susceptibility (T2*) contrast using multiple gradient echoes. AJNR Am J Neuroradiol. 2007;28(6):1093–4.
76. Vertinsky AT, Coenen VA, Lang DJ, Kolind S, Honey CR, Li D, et al. Localization of the subthalamic nucleus: optimization with susceptibility-weighted phase MR imaging. AJNR Am J Neuroradiol. 2009;30(9):1717–24.
77. Cuny E, Guehl D, Burbaud P, Gross C, Dousset V, Rougier A. Lack of agreement between direct magnetic resonance imaging and statistical determination of a subthalamic target: the role of electrophysiological guidance. J Neurosurg. 2002;97(3):591–7.
78. Andrade-Souza YM, Schwalb JM, Hamani C, Eltahawy H, Hoque T, Saint-Cyr J, et al. Comparison of three methods of targeting the subthalamic nucleus for chronic stimulation in Parkinson's disease. Neurosurgery 2005 56(2 Suppl):360–8; discussion 360–368.
79. Schlaier J, Schoedel P, Lange M, Winkler J, Warnat J, Dorenbeck U, et al. Reliability of atlas-derived coordinates in deep brain stimulation. Acta Neurochir. 2005;147(11):1175–80. discussion 1180.
80. Ashkan K, Blomstedt P, Zrinzo L, Tisch S, Yousry T, Limousin-Dowsey P, et al. Variability of the subthalamic nucleus: the case for direct MRI guided targeting. Br J Neurosurg. 2007;21(2):197–200.
81. Koike Y, Shima F, Nakamizo A, Miyagi Y. Direct localization of subthalamic nucleus supplemented by single-track electrophysiological guidance in deep brain stimulation Lead implantation: techniques and clinical results. Stereotact Funct Neurosurg. 2008;86(3):173–8.

82. Acar F, Miller JP, Berk MC, Anderson G, Burchiel KJ. Safety of anterior commissure-posterior commissure-based target calculation of the subthalamic nucleus in functional stereotactic procedures. Stereotact Funct Neurosurg. 2007;85(6):287–91.
83. Richter EO, Hoque T, Halliday W, Lozano AM, Saint-Cyr JA. Determining the position and size of the subthalamic nucleus based on magnetic resonance imaging results in patients with advanced Parkinson disease. J Neurosurg. 2004;100(3):541–6.
84. Zhu XL, Hamel W, Schrader B, Weinert D, Hedderich J, Herzog J, et al. Magnetic resonance imaging-based morphometry and landmark correlation of basal ganglia nuclei. Acta Neurochir. 2002;144(10):959–69. discussion 968–969.
85. Littlechild P, Varma TRK, Eldridge PR, Fox S, Forster A, Fletcher N, et al. Variability in position of the subthalamic nucleus targeted by magnetic resonance imaging and microelectrode recordings as compared to atlas co-ordinates. Stereotact Funct Neurosurg. 2003;80(1–4):82–7.
86. Alvarez-Linera J. 3T MRI: advances in brain imaging. Eur J Radiol. 2008;67(3):415–26.
87. Cheng CH, Huang HM, Lin HL, Chiou SM. 1.5T versus 3T MRI for targeting subthalamic nucleus for deep brain stimulation. Br J Neurosurg. 2014;28(4):467–70.
88. Boutet A, Gramer R, Steele CJ, Elias GJB, Germann J, Maciel R, et al. Neuroimaging technological advancements for targeting in functional neurosurgery. Curr Neurol Neurosci Rep. 2019;19(7):42.
89. Elias GJB, Germann J, Loh A, Boutet A, Taha A, Wong EHY, et al. Normative connectomes and their use in DBS. In: Connectomic Deep Brain Stimulation [Internet]. Elsevier; 2022 [cited 2021 Dec 22]. p. 245–74. Available from: https://linkinghub.elsevier.com/retrieve/pii/B9780128218617000142
90. Boutet A, Loh A, Chow CT, Taha A, Elias GJB, Neudorfer C, et al. A literature review of magnetic resonance imaging sequence advancements in visualizing functional neurosurgery targets. J Neurosurg. 2021 Nov;135(5):1445–58.
91. Coenen VA, Allert N, Madler B. A role of diffusion tensor imaging fiber tracking in deep brain stimulation surgery: DBS of the dentato-rubro-thalamic tract (drt) for the treatment of therapy-refractory tremor. Acta Neurochir. 2011;153(8):1579–85. discussion 1585.
92. Sporns O, Tononi G, Kötter R. The human connectome: a structural description of the human brain. PLoS Comput Biol. 2005;1(4):e42.
93. Riva-Posse P, Choi KS, Holtzheimer PE, Crowell AL, Garlow SJ, Rajendra JK, et al. A connectomic approach for subcallosal cingulate deep brain stimulation surgery: prospective targeting in treatment-resistant depression. Molecular Psychiatry [Internet]. 2017; Apr 11 [cited 2017 Aug 29]; Available from: http://www.nature.com/doifinder/10.1038/mp.2017.59
94. Schlaepfer TE, Bewernick BH, Kayser S, Mädler B, Coenen VA. Rapid effects of deep brain stimulation for treatment-resistant major depression. Biol Psychiatry. 2013;73:1204–12.
95. Coenen VA, Allert N, Paus S, Kronenbürger M, Urbach H, Mädler B. Modulation of the Cerebello-Thalamo-cortical network in thalamic deep brain stimulation for tremor: a diffusion tensor imaging study. Neurosurgery. 2014;75(6):657–70.
96. Butson CR, Cooper SE, Henderson JM, Wolgamuth B, McIntyre CC. Probabilistic analysis of activation volumes generated during deep brain stimulation. NeuroImage. 2011;54(3):2096–104.
97. Dembek TA, Roediger J, Horn A, Reker P, Oehrn C, Dafsari HS, et al. Probabilistic Sweetspots Predict Motor Outcome for DBS in Parkinson's Disease. Ann Neurol. 2019 Aug 3;ana.25567.
98. Nowacki A, Barlatey S, Al-Fatly B, Dembek T, Bot M, Green AL, et al. Probabilistic mapping reveals optimal stimulation site in essential tremor. Annals of Neurology [Internet]. 2022; [cited 2022 Mar 7];n/a(n/a). Available from: https://onlinelibrary.wiley.com/doi/abs/10.1002/ana.26324
99. Horn A, Reich M, Vorwerk J, Li N, Wenzel G, Fang Q, et al. Connectivity predicts deep brain stimulation outcome in Parkinson disease. Ann Neurol. 2017;82(1):67–78.

Overview of the Clinical Aspects of DBS

3

Oliver Flouty, Brian Dalm, and Andres M. Lozano

Overview and History of DBS

Brief History of Neurostimulation in Functional Neurosurgery

Electrical neurostimulation is a neurosurgical tool that was used to investigate and explore regions of the brain by select neurosurgical centers early in the twentieth century. Penfield and his team developed the "Montreal Procedure" in the 1930s where awake patients underwent exploratory electrical stimulation to help localize seizure onset zones and map eloquent areas prior to resection. The localization technique, however, was laborious and open to subjective interpretation [1]. A decade later, human stereotaxy was born when methodical human brain localization using cartesian coordinates was developed in 1947 by two independent groups. Expanding upon an earlier predecessor frame built for animal experimentation by Horsley and Clarke in 1908, Spiegel (neurologist) and Wycis (neurosurgeon) described the first human stereotactic apparatus to perform ablative surgeries labeled as "stereoencephalotomies" (Fig. 3.1). The Spiegel–Wycis frame was primarily designed for psychosurgery at the time [2]. In the same year, Tailarach

O. Flouty (✉)
University of South Florida, Department of Neurosurgery and Brain Repair, Tampa, FL, USA
e-mail: Oliver.flouty@usf.edu

B. Dalm
Ohio State University Wexner Medical Center, Department of Neurosurgery, Columbus, OH, USA

A. M. Lozano
Division of Neurosurgery, University Health Network and University of Toronto, Toronto, ON, Canada
e-mail: Andres.Lozano@uhnresearch.ca

A. Boutet, A. M. Lozano (eds.), *Magnetic Resonance Imaging in Deep Brain Stimulation*, https://doi.org/10.1007/978-3-031-16348-7_3

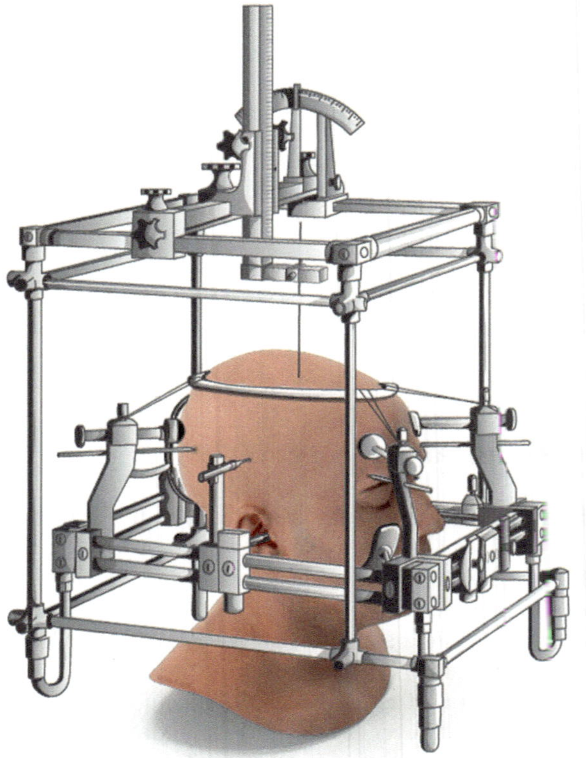

Fig. 3.1 An artist's adaptation of the earliest stereotactic frame built by Spiegel and Wycis in 1947

designed a unique stereotactic apparatus that was specifically intended to permit implantation of electrodes for recording and stimulation in epilepsy [3]. This heralded the era of stereotactic functional neurosurgery where frame-based stereotaxis allowed the use of neurophysiologic recordings in conjunction with electrical stimulation for assessing and exploring brain targets prior to lesioning. Subcortical mapping and electrical neurostimulation developed in parallel with lesioning and continued to gradually develop with chronic electrode implants, allowing for systematic and safe incremental lesioning until stimulation became a standalone modality for therapy.

While it is known that neuromodulation started first with psychosurgery followed by pain, epilepsy, and movement disorders, it is fair to say that linear narratives of the history of DBS provide an inadequate and an oversimplified version of the truth. It is therefore worth mentioning that technological advances in DBS were non-linear and history shows that slow advances took place in parallel as several groups were working with this technology separately and independently to treat various neuropsychological conditions. The groups at the time shared similar goals of safe lesioning yet they had a heterogenous outlook on innovation, media sensationalism, resources, and regulation. Their work often sprouted simultaneously in different regions of the world and mainly in Europe and the United States.

DBS for Psychosurgery

Chronic depth electrode implantation for stimulation and recording was proposed as early as the late 1940s and early 1950s. Among the earliest pioneers of chronic depth electrode implantation for recording and stimulation included Heath in New Orleans, Sems-Jacobson in Oslo, and Delgado in Connecticut. At that time, the earliest indication for stereotactic surgery was to treat psychiatric and behavioral disorders [4–7]. The surgeries were not standardized. Practitioners who included neurologists and neurobehaviorists often worked in isolation, and the questionable ethical grounds of their treatment protocols were open to interpretation [8]. Results were often subjective and lacked scientific rigor and transparency Systematic studies done subsequently failed to prove efficacy of DBS for psychosurgery and the field fell out of favor. At this time, DBS is still being practiced for psychiatric conditions, mainly for obsessive compulsive disorder (OCD). Yet, it is a minority of DBS indications, and outside OCD, this practice remains investigational.

DBS for Pain

DBS for pain started as early as the 1950s and underwent a surge in the 1970s primarily by two groups, Mazars and Hosobuchi in France and USA, respectively [9, 10]. Pain targets included sensory thalamus, internal capsule, and periventricular/periaqueductal gray [11–14]. Chronic subcortical stimulation for chronic pain using multi targeting of thalamus and periventricular gray became a popular procedure that Medtronic trademarked the term DBS in the mid-1970s. Functional practitioners reported that the surgeries were very effective. Unfortunately, clinical trials failed to show that DBS offers good efficacy for pain and therefore DBS for pain never took off or became a standard of care.

DBS for Epilepsy

DBS for epilepsy started at a later stage following investigational DBS for psychosurgery; however its adoption and progress did overlap with other indications including psychosurgery and pain. The original frame designed by Tailarach was specifically designed to allow chronic implantation of electrodes for recording and stimulation in epilepsy [3]. Over the course of the next two decades, other targets such as the cerebellum and the anterior nucleus of the thalamus were later introduced [15, 16]. The latter of which re-emerged several years later and more recently with showing progressive improvement of seizure control reaching up to 67% 3 years after DBS [17].

DBS for Movement Disorders

Among the earliest recorded frame-based functional procedures in movement disorder was a pallidotomy for Huntington chorea dating back to 1950, where electrical stimulation was used intraoperatively prior to lesioning [18]. The emergence of DBS for movement disorders, however, appeared later in the 1960s and followed DBS for psychosurgery, pain, and epilepsy [19, 20]. Microelectrode recording and stimulation of the ViM thalamus with high frequency stimulation to treat tremor in PD was recorded as early as 1963 by Albe-Fessard [21]. In the late 1960s, functional neurosurgery experienced a decline when Levodopa was introduced. Referring providers became reluctant to refer Parkinson's disease patients to neurosurgeons since the new drug was perceived as safe, effective, and inexpensive. Soon after its introduction, Levodopa quickly became the first-line treatment for PD and overshadowed functional procedures for 10 to 20 years. DBS re-emerged when many patients treated with levodopa became refractory to medical management and experienced significant side effects from their medications and disease progression. The earliest recorded permanent thalamic DBS implant was reported by Brice et al. in 1980 for secondary intention tremor associated with multiple sclerosis (MS) [22]. Seven years later, Benabid and his group in Grenoble, France, implanted a unilateral permanent thalamic DBS system in a patient suffering from essential tremor who had undergone contralateral Vim lesioning [23]. His collaborative and multidisciplinary approach, combined with a systematic analysis of efficacy, and the standardization of the surgical technique ushered a new era of modern DBS. Since then, DBS for movement disorders has been the dominant indication in the field.

Other Indications

DBS was also investigated for other indications including decreased level of consciousness starting in the late 1960s until the 1990s without gaining significant traction as the results were heterogenous and difficult to interpret and reproduce [24–26].

Regulation of DBS Implants

The FDA granted approval of thalamic DBS for treatment of tremor in 1997. Six years later, the FDA approved STN and GPi DBS to treat advanced medically uncontrolled PD. Until the FDA asserted authority over implantable medical devices in the 1970s, the design, fabrication, clinical testing, and marketing of neurostimulation hardware were relatively unregulated in the United States. A change in regulatory climate took place in 1976 when the US Congress passed the Medical Device Amendments and granted the FDA authority over all medical devices. The FDA was given the role of providing guidelines, oversight, and assurances of reasonable safety and effectiveness of devices under investigation prior to release in the medical field market. While regulating medical devices brought about an end to the era of unsupervised investigational use of DBS on one hand, it also increased patient safety, transparency of clinical efficacy, and minimized the practice of haphazard and unsafe human experimentation. It is also notable that increased regulation restricted research and slowed down innovation.

Today, approximately 15,000 DBS systems get implanted every year [27]. MRI-compatible closed-loop DBS systems nowadays are capable of sensing pathologic neurophysiological signatures and adapting its stimulation paradigm accordingly. The global market size was valued at 1.2 billion US dollars in 2020 and is projected to increase by 9% in 2028 [28]. Such growth seems to reflect (1) an increase in patient referrals as more and more neurologists open up to this treatment modality and (2) a renaissance in DBS for other conditions to include various ailments such as OCD, Tourette syndrome, morbid obesity, aggression, depression, and addiction.

Patient Selection and Referral

Most patients referred to neurosurgical evaluation come from a neurology clinic with a small minority coming from psychiatry. As with any surgical procedure, the key to optimizing outcomes starts with proper patient selection [29]. Those patients typically suffer from a movement disorder such as Parkinson's disease or tremor that had failed medical management either through medication side effects or motor fluctuations. Once all conservative measures are depleted, patients undergo neurosurgical evaluation, neuroimaging, neuropsychological evaluation, and evaluation at a multidisciplinary movement disorder conference [30].

Neurology Screening

All patients being considered for surgical intervention for a movement disorder should start their workup with a specialty trained movement disorder neurologist. It is critical to differentiate essential tremor from other common tremor syndromes or Parkinson's disease from disorders that can mimic Parkinson's such as multiple system atrophy as many of these other conditions are difficult to manage or respond poorly with DBS therapy. Additionally, prior to undergoing surgical intervention it is critical to ensure that all medical options have been thoroughly exhausted and that patients either cannot tolerate the medications secondary to side effects or have significant motor fluctuations. This includes both oral medications and, in some indications, injectable Botox. A thorough evaluation of previous medications is key since certain medications, such as neuroleptics, can induce a parkinsonian-like state that can be reversible with drug cessation.

Once the neurological diagnosis is confirmed and surgical consideration has been determined, patients start a series of steps to help determine whether DBS therapy may be an effective option in mitigating their symptoms. This typically involves utilizing standardized measurement tools to help score the severity of symptoms such as the Fahn–Tolosa–Marin tremor rating scale for essential tremor and the Unified Parkinson Disease Rating Scale (UPDRS) for Parkinson's disease. Patients will undergo videotaped examinations for later review at the movement disorder conference. For Parkinson's disease, the motor subsection of the UPDRS, section III, is used and patients are evaluated through a Levodopa challenge test where they are examined off medications and on medications. A UPDRS III score of greater than 30 is generally recommended off medications with a greater than 33% reduction in the on-medication state [31].

Neurosurgical Evaluation

The primary goal of the initial neurosurgical evaluation of potential DBS candidates is to verify correct diagnosis, verify that appropriate medical management has been pursued, evaluate for "red flags" to DBS surgery, and verify that the patient is an appropriate candidate to undergo a surgical procedure. Certain factors such as diabetes, cardiac risk factors, liver disease, kidney disease, or coagulopathies may have to be factored in to determine whether the risk of undergoing brain surgery outweighs the benefits of the operation. Additionally, this is a time where the surgeon can discuss with the patient the details of the operation, complications, and answer any questions that the patients will have about the surgery. A comprehensive neurological physical examination should be performed.

Neuropsychiatric Testing

All patients undergoing surgical consideration for Parkinson's disease should undergo neuropsychological evaluation. With regard to essential tremor, this tends to be more site-specific with no consensus that preoperative neuropsychological evaluation is mandatory. Movement disorder patients, particularly Parkinson patients, can have underlying psychiatric comorbidities such as depression and the incidence of mild cognitive impairment and dementia are higher in Parkinson patients. Additionally, these patients are at higher risk for further cognitive impairment following DBS surgery [32].

Neuroimaging

Preoperative MRI is critical to evaluate the patient-specific neuroanatomy. Brain tumors, previous strokes, ventriculomegaly, and cerebral atrophy can all be identified. If the diagnosis of Parkinson's disease is questioned, MRI imaging and other modalities, such as a dopamine tomography scan (DaT scan), can be utilized to assist and guide the diagnosis [33]. MRI is also critical as preoperative target planning of DBS lead placement is largely anatomical and high-quality MRI imaging is a key component that helps identify target structures and delineate neighboring anatomy for optimal direct and anatomical targeting.

Contraindications to Surgery

Generally, the usual contraindications to any surgery are applicable to DBS surgery. This can include cardiopulmonary disease, coagulopathies, advanced age, and significant medical comorbidities. More specifically, little to no response to the levodopa challenge test except in tremor dominant patients is a negative predictor for treatment success [34]. Cognitive impairment and dementia can be a contraindication but may need to be evaluated on a case-by-case basis. Red flags such as REM behavior sleep disorder, significant hypophonia, visual hallucinations, orthostasis, absence of anosmia, medication unresponsive freezing of gait, significant balance problems with a history of frequent falls, dysphagia, or dysarthria should also give pause before proceeding with DBS surgery [35].

Clinical Considerations and Target Selection

DBS for Essential Tremor

Essential tremor is a tremor of postural action that can affect multiple body parts including hands, head and neck, laryngeal muscles, and rarely the leg. It is familial in 50% of the cases with a bimodal age of onset of peaking during the second and sixth decade. Patients usually become aware of the disease when it starts involving the dominant hand and becomes more frustrating as the tremor spreads to the non-dominant hand with time. The typical tremor frequency is around 5–15 Hz and can have a high amplitude causing social embarrassment, interfering with the quality of the patients' life and activities of daily living such as eating, drinking, and writing. The tremor can be exacerbated by stress and stimulants such as caffeine. It can be relieved by alcohol, beta blockers, primidone, benzodiazepines and barbiturates. Fifty percent of patients do not respond to pharmacological therapy and may be considered for surgical candidacy [36].

Action tremor is a clinical diagnosis that should be differentiated from mild dystonic tremor especially if the patient complains of limb or neck pain with or without posturing. Task-specific tremor should also be differentiated such as writer's tremor. Parkinsonian tremor can mimic ET with action tremor (ET+). In such case, look for other mild symptoms of PD. Fortunately, DBS works for writer's tremor, dystonic tremor, and Parkinsonian tremor. Since essential tremor is a cerebellar disease, ataxia and gait imbalance are common, especially in older patients. Should a patient present with advanced age or impaired gait, consideration should be given to unilateral procedure to mitigate the risk of worsening stimulation-induced gait instability. Bilateral procedures can also increase the risk of dysarthria as well which might be disabling to some patients.

Common targets for ET include the ViM nucleus of the thalamus (Fig. 3.2) and Zona Incerta (also called the posterior subthalamic area or PSA) [36, 37]. Side effects of stimulation include transient paresthesia, which is often more pronounced with ZI DBS. When paresthesia is persistent at low voltages, think of posterior electrode placement in sensory thalamus, Vc. Such paresthesia typically involves the fingertips

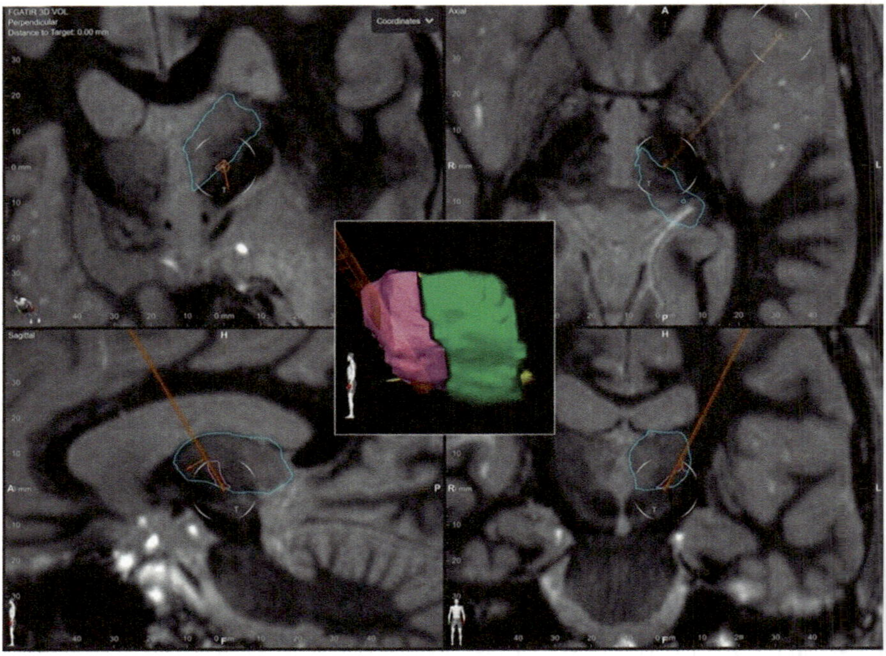

Fig. 3.2 Magnetic resonance imaging demonstrating a left-sided ViM DBS directional lead in the axial (right upper panel), sagittal (left lower panel), coronal (right lower panel), and perpendicular planes (left upper panel). The perpendicular plan denotes the plane perpendicular to the DBS lead. The cyan tracing denotes the outer circumference of the thalamus. The central panel demonstrates the relationship of the DBS lead contact with the left ViM nucleus (pink) and its proximity to the sensory thalamus, Vc (green). Figures were generated using the Elements software by Brainlab, Boston Scientific®

or the corner of the mouth and should alert the surgeon that the electrode is likely placed 2–3 mm posterior to ViM. Dysarthria is another side effect of ViM or ZI stimulation. It can result from activation of motor fibers within the corticospinal tract just lateral to the ViM nucleus. Typically, such a form of dysarthria does not adapt or suppress with time, and therefore should be differentiated from transient dysarthria with adaptation that typically improves spontaneously when given enough time. Such transient form of dysarthria is hypothesized to result from activation of cerebellothalamic fiber tracts responsible for coordination of speech. In addition to persistent stimulation-induced dysarthria, lateral placement of the electrode can also lead to facial pulling and muscle contractions due to current spread into the corticospinal fibers within the internal capsule. Anterior misplacement of the electrode will lead to diminished or absent tremor control. Ventral placement of the electrode can cause activation of the cerebellar fibers of the brachium conjunctivum medially, the internal capsule laterally, or the medial lemniscal pathway posteriorly. Activation of the cerebellar fibers can cause ataxia. Activation of the medial lemniscal pathway leads to low threshold contralateral paresthesia distributed over a large surface area of the body. This should be differentiated from paresthesia seen with Vc stimulation which typically requires higher voltages and is restricted to a small surface area of the contralateral body such as the corner of the mouth or the hand.

DBS for Idiopathic Parkinson's Disease

Idiopathic Parkinson's disease is a multisystem neurodegenerative disease affecting 0.6% of the population above 45 years of age and can increase by four to five times in people above the age of 65. Today, it is estimated that ten million individuals are affected worldwide. It is classically characterized by a triad of resting tremor, bradykinesia, and cogwheel rigidity. PD is diagnosed clinically and is characterized by the presence of two or more cardinal features. The disease is initially responsive to dopaminergic agents such as Levodopa. Over time, and as the disease progresses, some patients become resistant to medical management and can experience significant side effects from increased medication requirements.

It is important that an experienced movement disorder neurologist evaluates the patient prior to surgical referral as there are many other diseases that can mimic PD. Prior to consideration of DBS, PD should unequivocally be differentiated from PD mimickers such as dementia with Lewy bodies (DLB), progressive supra nuclear palsy (PSP), multiple system atrophy (MSA), corticobasal syndrome, and normal pressure hydrocephalus (NPH). Conditions that mimic PD can be ruled out by an experienced neurologist through an extensive history, clinical examination, and neuroimaging. PD mimickers can masquerade as PD during their early presentation. It is therefore crucial to consider surgical candidacy for PD no earlier than 5 years from disease onset.

DBS target selection for PD should result from a multidisciplinary discussion between the neurologist, neuropsychiatrist, neurosurgeon, and the movement disorder nurse. This discussion should review the patient's clinical presentation and examination as well as review all the pertinent screening investigations. The patient's candidacy and suitability for surgery should be reviewed and contraindications, if present, should be discussed. Classical targets to treat intractable PD include the subthalamic nucleus (STN) and the internal segment of globus pallidus (GPi). In cases of tremor dominant PD, ViM or caudal Zona Incerta (cZi) targeting can also be considered.

STN DBS

This target is typically recommended for patients with good cognitive reserve who are receiving a high dose of L-DOPA or dopamine agonists and experiencing significant side effects from the medical treatment. The STN is a very effective target in reducing tremor, bradykinesia, and rigidity. It can also help improve gait unsteadiness and freezing symptoms if they are responsive to dopaminergic medications. STN DBS is also effective in mitigating dyskinesia mostly through reducing the number of medications as drug dosage can be reduced by up to 50%, once therapy is initiated and stimulation parameters are optimized. STN DBS can occasionally cause cognitive and behavioral adverse effects. These side effects are more often observed with targeting of the anterior and medial portion of STN and can include apathy, disinhibition, and cognitive impairment. Contralateral paresthesia that does not habituate with time is a typical sign of posterior placement of the electrode and activation of the medial lemniscal fibers. Medial placement of the electrode can lead to current spread to the oculomotor nerve fibers leading to diplopia secondary to ipsilateral mono ocular medial deviation and rotation of the eye. Medial misplacement of the electrode can also lead to stimulation of the red nucleus as well which can cause nausea, discomfort, and sweating (Fig. 3.3). Contralateral tetanic contraction of the limbs and face or sustained dysarthria are typically seen with anterolateral placement of the electrode and stimulation of the corticospinal tract. Lateral placement of the electrode can engage frontal eye field fibers of the internal capsule causing contralateral bilateral gaze deviation which should be distinguished from the mono ocular findings seen with oculomotor fiber stimulation. Anterior

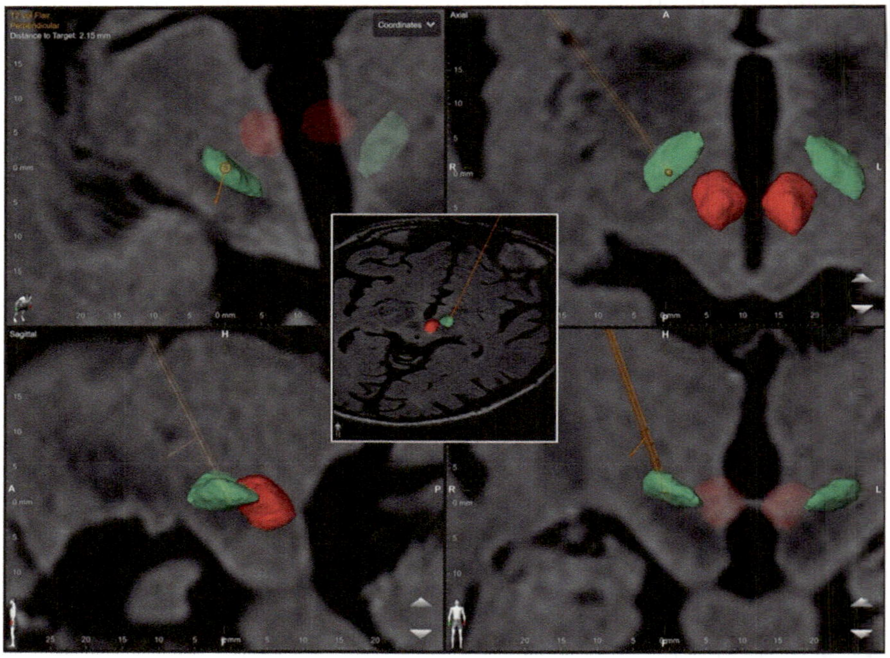

Fig. 3.3 Magnetic resonance imaging demonstrating a right-sided STN DBS directional lead in the axial (right upper panel), sagittal (left lower panel), coronal (right lower panel), and perpendicular planes (left upper panel). The perpendicular plan denotes the plane perpendicular to the DBS lead. Three dimensional models of STN and the red nucleus are depicted in green and red, respectively. The central panel demonstrates the relationship of the DBS lead contact with the STN nucleus. Figures were generated using the Elements software by Brainlab, Boston Scientific®

misplacement of the electrode can also be silent and leads to no effect on cardinal symptoms nor visible side effects with stimulation. Rarely, patients can experience autonomic symptoms such as flushing and sweating, and this can be a sign of hypothalamic stimulation seen with anteromedial misplacement of the electrode. Deep placement of the electrode will lead to stimulation of the SNr which is located ventral to STN. Observed effects of SNr stimulation can include akinesia and acute mood changes.

GPi DBS

This target is typically recommended to patients with cognitive dysfunction or mood disorder that is identified on the preoperative neuropsychological screening. GPi can also be considered for patients who suffer concomitant limb dystonia or gait disturbances that are not responsive to medications. Despite conflicting evidence, studies have advocated GPi as the better target in candidates harboring

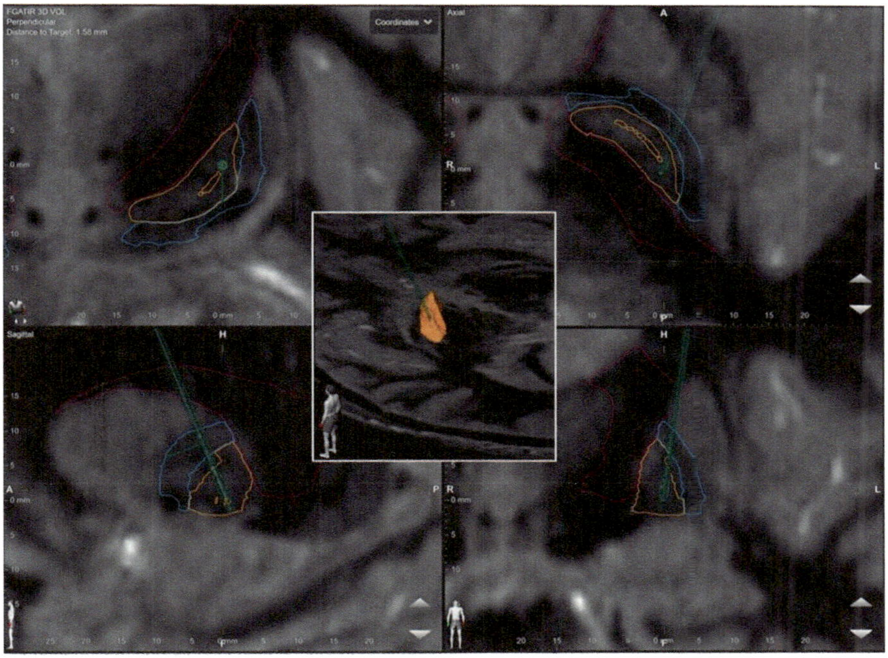

Fig. 3.4 Magnetic resonance imaging demonstrating a left-sided GPi DBS directional lead in the axial (right upper panel), sagittal (left lower panel), coronal (right lower panel), and perpendicular planes (left upper panel). The perpendicular plan denotes the plane perpendicular to the DBS lead. The cyan tracing denotes the internal capsule. The blue and orange tracings denote the external and internal segments of globus pallidus, respectively. The central panel demonstrates an oblique view showing the relationship of the DBS lead contact with the left GPi nucleus (orange) overlayed on an axial slice. Figures were generated using the Elements software by Brainlab, Boston Scientific®

cognitive or psychiatric concerns on preoperative screening. Studies have shown that GPi targeting is more forgiving when it comes to cognitive side effects profile. GPi DBS is therefore being increasingly targeted for elderly patients with cognitive and memory impairment given the target's relatively lower cognitive side effects morbidity when compared to STN. GPi DBS typically does not offer a reduction in medication dosing and patients still require the same medication dosage that was prescribed preoperatively and are expected to increase the medication doses as the disease progresses. The globus pallidus is located medial to the putamen, lateral to the internal capsule, and dorsal to the optic tract (Fig. 3.4). Effective electrode placement in the posterior third of the GPi will lead to reduction of parkinsonian symptoms. Observed stimulation-induced side effects can include muscle contractions if the electrode is placed medially and/or posteriorly to the effective target. Patients might experience flickering lights or phosphenes in the contralateral visual hemifield if the electrode is placed ventral to the effective target by activating the optic tract fibers. Lateral and anterior placement of the electrode can sometimes cause improvement in PD symptoms if the electrode is in the medial border of GPe. However, no observed improvement in PD symptoms is the common finding seen with anterior and lateral electrode misplacements.

ViM/cZi for Tremor-Dominant PD

Vim/cZi targeting can be considered when tremor is the sole poorly controlled symptom. The main side effects with targeting Vim and cZi are speech and balance impairment which is more commonly seen with bilateral targeting. These two targets are especially appealing in elderly patients with multiple comorbidities having poorly controlled unilateral dominant hand tremor due to low rate of complications with unilateral DBS implantation. As expected, drug dosage is usually stable after this operation. From a programming standpoint, Vim/Zi programming is typically less cumbersome when compared to GPi and especially STN DBS.

DBS for Dystonia

Dystonia is a disorder of involuntary repetitive patterned movements caused by concurrent painful contractions of agonist and antagonist muscle groups that can involve the limbs or axial skeleton. It can be triggered by voluntary action and is associated with painful overflow muscle activation. There are multiple subtypes and classifications of dystonia. The success of DBS for dystonia is dependent on key factors which include the dystonia distribution, associated symptoms, structural alterations of the brain, as well as age of onset, genetics, and body distribution. Patients failing medical management can be considered for DBS. Of note, there are no clear DBS indications under validated criteria for symptoms such as severity scores or pharmacological treatment cut-offs. It is therefore important to identify the target symptoms amenable to DBS therapy and define expectations early when considering DBS. Those discussions should be made directly with the patient. In case of cognitively impaired patients or children, caregivers and parents should be involved. It is important to rule out triggering factors such as abrupt changes in medication dosing or infections and to make sure treatable causes are excluded. Medical management includes anticholinergic agents, benzodiazepines, dopaminergic medication, gabapentin, and Botox injections. Typically, fixed dystonic posture does not improve with DBS. A classical workup includes genetic tests, blood tests to exclude metabolic disorders, and MRI. DBS is most effective against primary isolated dystonia such as cervical dystonia and blepharospasm. Secondary dystonia is more complex to treat as it may be associated with a variety of brain disorders including various neurological conditions and trauma. Secondary dystonia is, therefore, less responsive to DBS. Unlike tremor, dystonia symptoms take time to respond to DBS and sometimes can take weeks and up to months for the stimulation to be optimized and symptoms to be relieved. Common stimulation-induced side effects include dysarthria and imbalance. If the electrode is placed too deep, it can induce flickering lights secondary to activation of the optic tract. Motor contraction of the face and limbs is an indication of activation of the corticospinal fibers in the internal capsule and can indicate medial and/or posterior placement of the electrode.

DBS for Epilepsy

Epilepsy is a disorder of abnormal neuronal synchrony that can be controlled with antiepileptic drugs. While the vast majority of seizures are treated medically, 30% of adults with epilepsy do not achieve seizure freedom with medical management and are therefore considered for surgical candidacy. Surgical treatment of epilepsy involves the excision of the ictal onset zone or disconnecting it from the surrounding network. If surgical resection or disconnection is not appropriate, patients may be considered for neurostimulation treatment. The most widely used target for neurostimulation in patients suffering from drug resistant epilepsy (DRE) is the anterior nucleus of the thalamus (ANT). Other targets for DRE include the centromedian thalamic nucleus (CMTN), hippocampus, basal ganglia, and cerebellum. Adverse effects from ANT stimulation include stimulation-induced seizures, paresthesia, depression, and memory impairment. ANT DBS leads traverse the lateral ventricles and therefore increase the theoretical chance of CSF leak. ANT DBS can decrease seizure frequency with a sequential improvement in seizure control from 40% after 1 year and reaching up to 70% at 3 years following DBS [17].

DBS for Other Indications

DBS has been investigated for various other neurological conditions and psychiatric disorders including Huntington's disease, disorders of consciousness, depression, anorexia nervosa, pain, aggression, morbid obesity, and Alzheimer's disease. The collective literature on these topics is too limited, many of the indications are still experimental, and selection criteria are still not established. Those topics are beyond the scope of this book, and therefore will not be further discussed.

Surgical Considerations

Intraoperative Considerations

Deep brain stimulation can be performed in a multitude of ways. Generally, the choice for how to perform the operation is site-specific and is based on surgeon's preferences. The traditional standard for DBS surgery is to perform the operations awake with a stereotactic frame, intraoperative microelectrode recordings, and awake stimulation testing. Additionally, frameless options are available as well as asleep techniques that can be performed entirely in the MRI suite or in the OR with intraoperative CT capabilities. The newest addition to deep brain stimulation has been the introduction of robot-assisted lead placement. In this scenario, the robot replaces the traditional ring and arc used to guide lead placement.

Postoperative Considerations

Postoperatively, all DBS patients are monitored in the hospital. This should occur in a setting where continuous vital sign monitoring with telemetry is available. Postoperative blood pressure monitoring is essential with normotensive parameters to limit the risk of postop hemorrhage. Additionally, postoperative imaging, such as a CT scan or MRI, should be obtained in a delayed fashion of around 6 h to evaluate for delayed postoperative bleeding complications and evaluate electrode positioning. Headache is a common postoperative complaint following DBS surgery and can be easily managed with acetaminophen or low dose opioids. If awake DBS surgery is employed, this generally utilizes primarily intravenous anesthetic agents which can significantly increase the chance for postoperative nausea. Scopolamine patches and antiemetics may need to be employed to decrease any episodes of emesis which can increase intracranial pressure and increase the risk for postoperative hemorrhage.

Future Directions and Innovations

We hope that in the future, big data collection and increased analytic capability will help clinicians choose and perhaps explore optimal targets and stimulation parameters for each individual patient based on their demographic and neuroimaging data. Furthermore, we will be able to stratify patients according to risk and use mathematical models to better predict the success of surgery, clinical outcomes, and side effects of stimulation based on the patient's clinical characteristics and specific measures derived from neuroimaging and neurophysiology data.

As the technology continues to develop, we anticipate improvement in hardware design, safety, closed-loop paradigms, and targeting by leveraging increased computing power, artificial intelligence, and improved quality of image acquisition. Improvement in hardware design can include improvements in electrode density with increasing number of electrode contacts allowing increased control over current spread through better control of volume of tissue activated (VTA) and current steering. As batteries continue to advance, IPGs will be able to have an improved lifetime and faster recharging or potentially energy harvesting capabilities. Improvement in safety measures could include improved MRI compatibility and privacy to protect users from hackers and potential "brain jacking." IPG improvement may also include the miniaturization and cranialization of the computerized generator. Such an advancement may lead to the total elimination of extension cables or second stage operations. IPGs will have increased control over waveform features and deliver independent currents and frequencies via different contacts while being able to simultaneously record from independent feedback sites. Those sites can include electrode contacts in the vicinity or far away from the stimulation site or from EMG data to improve upon closed-loop and adaptive capabilities. Such complex systems may depend on improved artificial intelligence algorithms mixed with improved computing power to provide fast online adaptation. Bluetooth capabilities will allow better chronic testing and experimentation and potentially the capability of open-source programming to deliver individualized stimulation/sensing paradigms. Advances in frameless technology including robot-assisted electrode placement and MRI-guided implantation as well as the introduction of mixed reality platforms could 1 day eliminate the need for frame placement and complex targeting and improve upon the efficiency of DBS surgery and its workflow. Advances in neuroimaging can also help better targeting via enhanced anatomic resolution, and when mixed with AI algorithms, can help automatically reconstruct DBS leads and seamlessly segment individual brains, as well as allow us to identify target "sweet-spots" from large retrospective datasets and perhaps predict stimulation settings, suggest active contacts, and predict outcomes and side effect probabilities.

Taken together, such future improvements will immensely help improve patient outcomes and break barriers to progress by accelerating advancements in neuroscience and ultimately help neurosurgeon-scientists push the envelope of neural-network science and help provide improved patient-specific treatments.

References

1. Penfield W. Epilepsy and surgical therapy. Arch Neurol Psychiatr. 1936;36(3):449–84.
2. Spiegel EA, Wycis HT, Marks M, Lee AJ. Stereotaxic apparatus for operations on the human brain. Science. 1947;106(2754):349–50. https://doi.org/10.1126/science.106.2754.349.
3. Talairach J, Bancaud J, Bonis A, Szikla G, Tournoux P. Functional stereotaxic exploration of epilepsy. Confin Neurol. 1962;22:328–31. https://doi.org/10.1159/000104378.
4. Pool JL. Psychosurgery in older people. J Am Geriatr Soc. 1954;2(7):456–66. https://doi.org/10.1111/j.1532-5415.1954.tb02138.x.
5. Delgado JM, Mark V, Sweet W, Ervin F, Weiss G, Bach YRG, et al. Intracerebral radio stimulation and recording in completely free patients. J Nerv Ment Dis. 1968;147(4):329–40. https://doi.org/10.1097/00005053-196810000-00001.
6. Sem-Jacobsen CW. Depth-electrographic observations in psychotic patients: a system related to emotion and behavior. Acta Psychiatr Scand Suppl. 1959;34(136):412–6. https://doi.org/10.1111/j.1600-0447.1959.tb07829.x.

7. Heath RG. Correlations between levels of psychological awareness and physiological activity in the central nervous system. Psychosom Med. 1955;17(5):383–95.
8. Baumeister AA. The Tulane electrical brain stimulation program a historical case study in medical ethics. J Hist Neurosci. 2000;9(3):262–78. https://doi.org/10.1076/jhin.9.3.262.1787.
9. Mazars G, Merienne L, Cioloca C. Treatment of certain types of pain with implantable thalamic stimulators. Neurochirurgie. 1974;20(2):117–24.
10. Mazars G, Merienne L, Ciolocca C. Intermittent analgesic thalamic stimulation. Preliminary note. Rev Neurol (Paris). 1973;128(4):273–9.
11. Hosobuchi Y, Adams JE, Linchitz R. Pain relief by electrical stimulation of the central gray matter in humans and its reversal by naloxone. Science. 1977;197(4299):183–6. https://doi.org/10.1126/science.301658.
12. Adams JE, Hosobuchi Y, Fields HL. Stimulation of internal capsule for relief of chronic pain. J Neurosurg. 1974;41(6):740–4. https://doi.org/10.3171/jns.1974.41.6.0740.
13. Richardson DE, Akil H. Pain reduction by electrical brain stimulation in man. Part 1: acute administration in periaqueductal and periventricular sites. J Neurosurg. 1977;47(2):178–83. https://doi.org/10.3171/jns.1977.47.2.0178.
14. Richardson DE, Akil H. Pain reduction by electrical brain stimulation in man. Part 2: chronic self-administration in the periventricular gray matter. J Neurosurg. 1977;47(2):184–94. https://doi.org/10.3171/jns.1977.47.2.0184.
15. Cooper I, Upton A, Amin I. Reversibility of chronic neurologic deficits. Some effects of electrical stimulation of the thalamus and internal capsule in man. Stereotact Funct Neurosurg. 1980;43(3–5):244–58.
16. Upton A, Cooper I, Springman M, Amin I. Suppression of seizures and psychosis of limbic system origin by chronic stimulation of anterior nucleus of the thalamus. Int J Neurol. 1985;19:223–30.
17. Fisher R, Salanova V, Witt T, Worth R, Henry T, Gross R, et al. Electrical stimulation of the anterior nucleus of thalamus for treatment of refractory epilepsy. Epilepsia. 2010;51(5):899–908. https://doi.org/10.1111/j.1528-1167.2010.02536.x.
18. Spiegel EA, Wycis HT. Pallidothalamotomy in chorea. Arch Neurol Psychiatr. 1950;64(2):295–6.
19. Sem-Jacobsen CW. Depth electrographic stimulation and treatment of patients with Parkinson's disease including neurosurgical technique. Acta Neurol Scand Suppl. 1965;13(Pt 1):365–77. https://doi.org/10.1111/j.1600-0404.1965.tb01899.x.
20. Hariz MI, Blomstedt P, Zrinzo L. Deep brain stimulation between 1947 and 1987: the untold story. Neurosurg Focus. 2010;29(2):E1. https://doi.org/10.3171/2010.4.Focus10106.
21. Albe Fessard D, Arfel G, Guiot G, Derome P, Dela H, Korn H, et al. Characteristic electric activities of some cerebral structures in man. Ann Chir. 1963;17:1185–214.
22. Brice J, McLellan L. Suppression of intention tremor by contingent deep-brain stimulation. Lancet. 1980;1(8180):1221–2. https://doi.org/10.1016/s0140-6736(80)91680-3.
23. Benabid AL, Pollak P, Louveau A, Henry S, de Rougemont J. Combined (Thalamotomy and stimulation) stereotactic surgery of the VIM thalamic nucleus for bilateral Parkinson disease. Stereotact Funct Neurosurg. 1987;50(1–6):344–6. https://doi.org/10.1159/000100803.
24. Katayama Y, Tsubokawa T, Yamamoto T, Hirayama T, Miyazaki S, Koyama S. Characterization and modification of brain activity with deep brain stimulation in patients in a persistent vegetative state: PaiŽ related late positive component of cerebral evoked potential. Pacing Clin Electrophysiol. 1991;14
25. Tsubokawa T, Yamamoto T, Katayama Y, Hirayama T, Maejima S, Moriya T. Deep-brain stimulation in a persistent vegetative state: follow-up results and criteria for selection of candidates. Brain Inj. 1990;4(4):315–27. https://doi.org/10.3109/02699059009026185.
26. Yamamoto T, Katayama Y. Deep brain stimulation therapy for the vegetative state. Neuropsychol Rehabil. 2005;15(3–4):406–13. https://doi.org/10.1080/09602010443000353.
27. Lee DJ, Lozano CS, Dallapiazza RF, Lozano AM. Current and future directions of deep brain stimulation for neurological and psychiatric disorders. J Neurosurg. 2019;131(2):333–42. https://doi.org/10.3171/2019.4.Jns181761.

28. Research GV. Deep brain stimulation devices market size, share & trends analysis report by product (Single Channel, dual-channel), by application, by end-use, by region, and segment forecasts, 2021–2028. Deep Brain Stimulation Devices Market Report 2021:1–164.
29. Katz M, Kilbane C, Rosengard J, Alterman RL, Tagliati M. Referring patients for deep brain stimulation: an improving practice. Arch Neurol. 2011;68(8):1027–32. https://doi.org/10.1001/archneurol.2011.151.
30. Ford PJ, Kubu CS. Stimulating debate: ethics in a multidisciplinary functional neurosurgery committee. J Med Ethics. 2006;32(2):106–9. https://doi.org/10.1136/jme.200X.013151.
31. Defer GL, Widner H, Marié RM, Rémy P, Levivier M. Core assessment program for surgical interventional therapies in Parkinson's disease (CAPSIT-PD). Mov Disord. 1999;14(4):572–84. https://doi.org/10.1002/1531-8257(199907)14:4<572::aid-mds1005>3.0.cc;2-c.
32. Nicoletti A, Luca A, Baschi R, Cicero CE, Mostile G, Davì M, et al. Incidence of mild cognitive impairment and dementia in Parkinson's disease: the Parkinson's disease cognitive impairment study. Front Aging Neurosci. 2019;11:21. https://doi.org/10.3389/fnagi.2019.00021.
33. de la Fuente-Fernández R. Role of DaTSCAN and clinical diagnosis in Parkinson disease. Neurology. 2012;78(10):696–701. https://doi.org/10.1212/WNL.0b013e318248e520.
34. Welter ML, Houeto JL, Tezenas du Montcel S, Mesnage V, Bonnet AM, Pillon B, et al. Clinical predictive factors of subthalamic stimulation in Parkinson's disease. Brain. 2002;125(Pt 3):575–83. https://doi.org/10.1093/brain/awf050.
35. Okun MS, Fernandez HH, Rodriguez RL, Foote KD. Identifying candidates for deep brain stimulation in Parkinson's disease: the role of the primary care physician. Geriatrics. 2007;62(5):18–24.
36. Flora ED, Perera CL, Cameron AL, Maddern GJ. Deep brain stimulation for essential tremor: a systematic review. Mov Disord. 2010;25(11):1550–9. https://doi.org/10.1002/mds.23195.
37. Blomstedt P, Stenmark Persson R, Hariz G-M, Linder J, Fredricks A, Häggström B, et al. Deep brain stimulation in the caudal zona incerta versus best medical treatment in patients with Parkinson's disease: a randomised blinded evaluation. J Neurol Neurosurg Psychiat. 2018;89(7):710–6. https://doi.org/10.1136/jnnp-2017-317219.

Preoperative Planning of DBS Surgery with MRI

4

Aaron Loh, Clement T. Chow, Aida Ahrari, Kâmil Uludağ, Sriranga Kashyap, Harith Akram, and Ludvic Zrinzo

Introduction

The success of deep brain stimulation (DBS) is largely dependent on the accurate engagement of target structures. The preoperative planning of surgery—in which the target is delineated, and the trajectory of the DBS lead is decided upon—is therefore essential in maximizing therapeutic outcomes (Fig. 4.1). Traditionally, planning was based on indirect targeting methods. This technique estimates the location of targets in relation to fixed and identifiable anatomical landmarks and was initially adopted as DBS targets could not be visualized on ventriculography or CT [1]. However, indirect targeting does not sufficiently account for interindividual variability in the location of target structures [1, 2]. To improve DBS targeting accuracy, indirect targeting methods were coupled with additional techniques such as intraoperative microelectrode recordings and intraoperative stimulation testing in awake patients [3]. However, these methods are associated with increased operating times and require an increasing number of passes through the brain parenchyma, increasing the risk of intra- and postoperative complications [4].

A. Loh (✉) · C. T. Chow · A. Ahrari · K. Uludağ · S. Kashyap
University Health Network, Toronto, ON, Canada
e-mail: aaron.loh@mail.utoronto.ca; clem.chow@mail.utoronto.ca; aida.ahrari@mail.utoronto.ca; kamil.uludag@rmp.uhn.ca; sriranga.kashyap@rmp.uhn.ca

H. Akram · L. Zrinzo
Functional Neurosurgery Unit, Department of Clinical and Movement Neurosciences, University College London, Queen Square Institute of Neurology, London, UK

The National Hospital for Neurology and Neurosurgery, London, UK
e-mail: harith.akram@ucl.ac.uk; l.zrinzo@ucl.ac.uk

A. Boutet, A. M. Lozano (eds.), *Magnetic Resonance Imaging in Deep Brain Stimulation*, https://doi.org/10.1007/978-3-031-16348-7_4

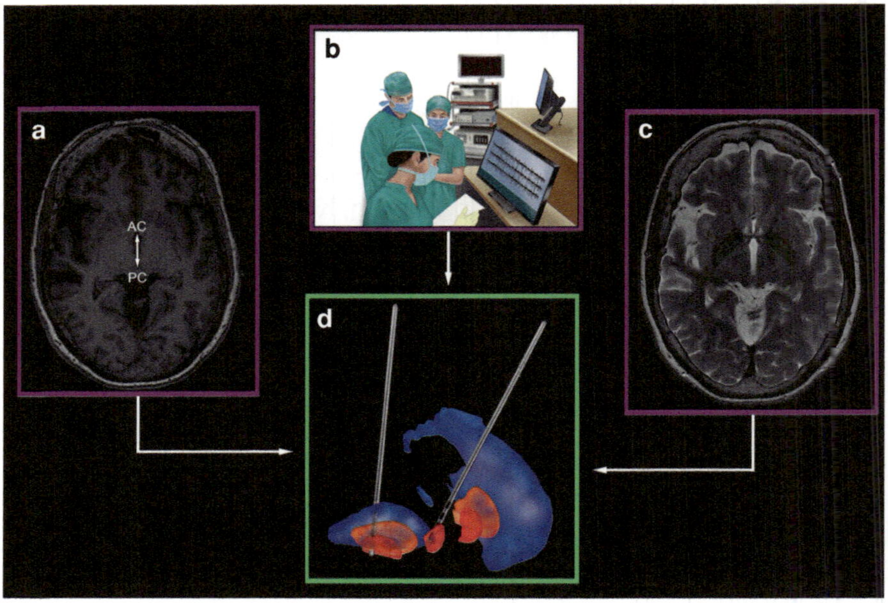

Fig. 4.1 DBS targeting strategies. A schematic of typical strategies employed in DBS lead placement (D), demonstrating indirect targeting with AC-PC fiducials (**a**), indirect targeting in addition to intraoperative MER (**b**), and direct targeting based on the direct visualization of target nuclei (**c**). Abbreviations: *AC-PC* anterior commissure-posterior commissure, *DBS* deep brain stimulation, *MER* microelectrode recordings

Routine brain MRI sequences acquired with standard field strengths (i.e., 1.5 or 3 Tesla) and acquisition parameters can have shortcomings in visualizing DBS targets [5]. However, with advances in stereotactic frames, MRI hardware, and pulse sequences, the direct visualization of certain structures, such as the subthalamic nucleus (STN), has replaced indirect targeting methods for preoperative planning at certain centers [4, 6]. Nonetheless, structures such as the thalamic nuclei remain challenging to visualize directly and continue to require indirect targeting [7]. To address this, novel MRI techniques have been developed and existing sequences have been optimized to improve the delineation of common DBS targets. It is important to note, however, that the ideal MRI sequence for DBS planning is not simply the technique that provides the greatest visibility of target structures. To maximize clinical translatability, it is crucial that the sequence is simple to implement, versatile (e.g., could be used for multiple targets and/or postoperative imaging), can be obtained with standard hardware and software, can be performed relatively quickly, provides sufficient contrast, and has minimal spatial or geometrical distortion.

Herein, we summarize and evaluate MRI sequences that have been used to improve the visualization of common DBS targets, highlight existing limitations, and discuss the potential future of DBS target planning.

Methods

Search

Studies with clinically used field strengths (i.e., 1.5 T or 3 T MRI) were identified following a comprehensive MEDLINE database search (December 2021) with a search strategy terms related to "Magnetic Resonance Imaging" and "Deep Brain Stimulation" and the most common neurosurgical targets, specifically a combination of exploded MeSH and free-text terms that comprised: (exp Magnetic Resonance Imaging OR (MRI OR magnetic resonance imag*).kw,tw.) AND (exp Electric Stimulation Therapy OR (stimulat* OR DBS).kw,tw.) AND (exp limbic system, OR exp. subthalamus, OR exp. thalamus) OR (STN OR subthal* OR thalam* OR GPi OR GPe OR globus pallidus).kw,tw.). A summary of all identified studies can be seen in Table 4.1.

Sequence Evaluation

Studies performed using "clinical" (i.e., 1.5 T or 3 T MRI) field strengths were assessed and scored using a weighted decision matrix on nominal or ordinal scales (Table 4.2; Fig. 4.2). The criteria assessed were: (A) whether it was described as the optimal sequence from its respective study (0 = no; 1 = yes), (B) described quality when used for direct stereotactic targeting (1 = average; 2 = good; 3 = excellent), (C) sample size scanned (1 = 1–10; 2 = 11–20; 3 = ≥ 21 participants), (D) whether diseased populations were scanned (0 = no; 1 = yes), (E) whether the sequence was performed on healthy controls (0 = no; 1 = yes), (F) number of sequences compared with (0 = none; 1 = 2–3; 2 = ≥ 4 sequences), and G) whether exogenous contrast or pre-/post-processing was required (1 = no; 0 = yes). Scores were summed to identify the most promising sequences for direct visualization of STN, GPi, and thalamic nuclei.

Table 4.1 Studies aiming to improve direct MRI visualization of DBS targets

	Study	Field Strength (T)	Sequences	Imaged Population (n)
Subthalamic nucleus	Thaker (2021)	3	Coronal GRE	PD (31), ET (7)
	Yu (2021)	3	QSM	PD (10)
	Morshita (2019)	1.5	T1w, FGATIR	PD (2), ET (3), Holmes (2)
	Rashid (2019)	1.5	IR, SPGR + C, SPGR	PD (8), ET (2), H (1)
	Bus (2018)	3	T1w, T2w, SWI	PD (45)
	Milchenko (2018)	3	Cube T2w, FLAIR 3D MPRAGE, 3D SPACE	PD (56)
	Rasouli (2018)	3	3D T2w FSE, T2w* multi-echo GRE / QSM	PD (122)
	Nowacki (2018)	3	T2w multi-echo FSE	PD (46)
	Alkamade (2017)	1.5	FLAWS	H (11)
	Zerroug (2016)	1.5	WAIR	PD (156)
	van Laar (2016)	1.5, 3	T2w TSE	PD (3)
	Verhagen (2016)	1.5	T2w TSE, 3D TSE	PD (14)
	Senova (2016)	1.5, 3	T1w, T2w, 3D SPACE FLAIR (3 T)	PD (10)
	Longhi (2015)	1, 3	T1w + T2w	PD (20)
	Lv (2015)	3	3D T2w DRIVE CLEAR, T1w, T2w*, T2w FLAIR, SWI	H (134)
	Xiao (2015)	3	T1w, T2w*, T1w–T2w*	PD (15)
	Sarkar (2015)	1.5	T2w FSE, FSTIR	H (12), PD (12)
	Heo (2015)	3	3D FLAIR, 2D T2w*-FFE, T2w-TSE	PD (20)
	Bériault (2014)	1.5	T1w-Gd and T1w + SWI + TOF	PD (21)
	Nagahama (2014)	3	T2w SWAN, T2w* GRE, T2w FSE	N/A (6)
	Lefranc (2014)	3	T2w SWAN	PD (8)
	Xiao (2015)	3	T1w, T2w*, phase image, R2*, FLASH	PD (10)
	Houshmand (2014)	3	T2w	PD (58)
	Deistung (2013)	3	MPRAGE	H (9)
	Liu (2013)	3	T2w, T2w*, R2*, phase, SWI	H (10), PD (8)
	Kerl (2012)	3	T2w FLAIR, T1w MPRAGE, T2w* FLASH2D, T2w SPACE, SWI	H (9)
	Patil (2012)	3	T1w	PD (20)
	Xiao (2012)	3	FLASH	H (4), PD (2)
	Ben-Haim et al. (2011)	1.5	FSE-IR, FSE-IR SPGR	PD (81)
	Cho (2010)	1.5, 3	T2w* GRE	H (11), PD (1)
	O'Gorman (2011)	1.5	T2w FSE, PDW FSE, SWI, PSIR, T2w*, DESPOT1, DESPOT2, IR-FSPGR	H (9), PD (10)
	Shen (2009)	1.5	T2w	H (122)
	Stancanello (2008)	3	T1w GRE, T2w FSE	H (10)
	Kitajima (2008)	3	T2w FSE, FSTIR	H (24)
	Elolf (2007)	3	Multi-echo FLASH, TSE	H (16)
	Ishimori (2007)	1.5	3D FSE	H (3), PD (2)
	Ashkan (2007)	1.5	T2w	PD (29)
	Slavin (2006)	3	T2w FSE	PD (13)
	Hariz (2003)	1.5	T2w	PD (N/A)
	Starr (2002)	1.5	T2w FSE, GRE	PD (76)

Table 4.1 (continued)

	Study	Field Strength (T)	Sequences	Imaged Population (n)
Globus pallidus	Yu (2021)	3	QSM	PD (10)
	Maruyama (2019)	3	PDW, T2w	H (12)
	Grewal (2018)	3	FGATIR	Epilepsy (1)
	Bender (2017)	3	MPRAGE	H (9)
	Zerroug (2016)	1.5	WAIR	PD (156)
	Jiltsova (2016)	1.5	STIR, T1w MPRAGE	Epilepsy (15)
	Ide (2015)	3	QSM	PD (19), H (41)
	Möttönen (2015)	3	STIR	Epilepsy (5)
	Duchin (2012)	1.5	T1w, T2w TSE	PD (12)
	Vassal (2012)	1.5	WAIR	PD (13), ET (7)
	Bender (2011)	3	3D MPRAGE	H (6)
	Yamada (2010)	1.5	STIR + DTI	H (10)
	Deoni (2007)	1.5	DESPOT1, DESPOT2	H (4)
	Spiegelmann (2006)	1.5, 3	FSE	ET (11)
	Hirabayashi (2002)	1.0	T1w SE	PD (48)
	Alterman (1999)	1.5	FSE/IR	MRT (17)
Thalamus	Morrison (2021)	3	PD	ET (2)
	Middlebrooks (2021	3	EDGE-MICRA	H (1)
	Nome (2020)	1.5, 3	T1w 3D	Epilepsy (18)
	Li (2019)	3	GRE 3D + QSM, T1w 3D, T2w 2D	PD (5), DYS (4), SCZ (3)
	Beaumont (2019)	1.5	FLAWS	H (12)
	Grewal (2018)	3	FGATIR HR, MPRAGE HR, MPRAGE	Epilepsy (1)
	Ide (2017)	3	PADRE, SWI, T2w	PD (20)
	Zerroug (2016)	1.5	WAIR	PD (156)
	Nowacki (2015)	3	T1w MPRAGE + Gd, MDEFT	PD, DYS (13)
	Buentjen (2013)	3	MPRAGE, TSE	H (6)
	Liu (2013)	3	T2w	H (10), PD (8)
	Nölte (2012)	3	FLAIR, T2w* SPACE, T2w* FLASH 2D, T2w* FLASH 2D-HB SWI	H (90)
	O'Gorman (2011)	1.5	T2w FSE, PDW FSE, SWI, PSIR, T2w* mapping, DESPOT1, IR-FSPGR	H (90)
	Sudhyadhom (2009)	3	T1w 3D MPRAGE, T2w 3D FLAIR, T1w 3D FGATIR	PD (1), ET (2)
	Pinsker (2008)	1.5	FSE-IR, T1w MPRAGE	DYS (23)
	Deichmann (2004)	1.5, 3	3D T1w MDEFT	H (7)
	Starr (1999)	1.5	T2w SE	H (51)

Sixty-four studies providing optimized sequences and post-processing methods for enhanced MRI visualization were included. Magnetic field strength, sequences as well as the population included are detailed. Abbreviations: *2/3D* two–/three-dimensional, *C* contrast, *CLEAR* constant level appearance, *DESPOT1/2* driven equilibrium single pulse observation of T1/2, *DRIVE* driven equilibrium RF reset pulse, *DTI* diffusion tensor imaging; *DYS* dystonia, *ET* essential tremor, *FFE* fast field echo, *EDGE-MICRA* edge-enhancing gradient echo-multi-image co-registration and averaging scan, *FGATIR* fast gray matter acquisition T1w inversion recovery, *FLAIR* fluid-attenuated inversion recovery, *FLASH* fast low angle shot, *FLASH2D-HB* FLASH2D with a high bandwidth of 200 kHz, *FLAWS* fluid and white matter suppression, *FSE* fast spin echo, *FSPGR* fast spoiled gradient echo, *FSTIR* short-T1 inversion recovery, *Gd* gadolinium, *GRE* gradient echo, *H* healthy,

(continued)

Table 4.1 (continued)

Holmes Holmes tremor, *IR* inversion recovery, *MDEFT* modified driven equilibrium Fourier transform, *MPRAGE* magnetization-prepared rapid gradient echo, *PADRE* phase difference-enhanced imaging, *PD* Parkinson's disease, *PDW* proton density-weighted; *PSIR* phase-sensitive inversion recovery, *QSM* quantitative susceptibility mapping, *R2** R2* mapping, *SCZ* schizophrenia, *SE* spin echo, *SPACE* turbo spin echo sequence variation, *SPGR* spoiled gradient recalled echo, *STIR* short-T1 inversion recovery, *SWAN* susceptibility-weighted angiography, *SWI* susceptibility-weighted imaging, *T* tesla, *T1w* T1-weighted, *T2w* T2-weighted, *TSE* turbo spin echo, *TOF* time-of-flight, *WAIR* white matter attenuated inversion recovery

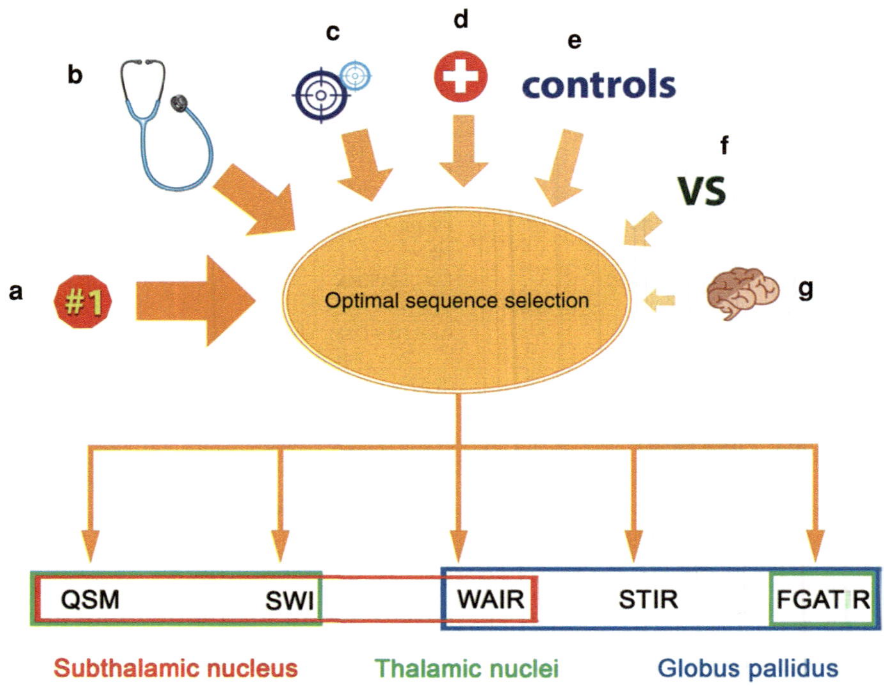

Fig. 4.2 Optimized sequences for improved visualization of common DBS targets. For each target (i.e., STN, GP, or thalamus), studies performed using "clinical" (i.e., 1.5 T or 3 T MRI) field strengths were assessed and scored using a weighted decision matrix on nominal or ordinal scales. The criterion included: (**a**) optimal sequence parameter from its respective study (0 = no; 1 = yes), (**b**) described quality when used for direct stereotactic targeting (1 = average; 2 = good; 3 = excellent), (**c**) sample size scanned (1 = 1–10; 2 = 11–20; 3 = ≥ 21 participants), (**d**) diseased populations scanned (0 = no; 1 = yes), (**e**) sequence was compared to controls (0 = no; 1 = yes), (**f**) number of sequences compared with (0 = none; 1 = 2–3; 2 = ≥ 4 sequences), and (**g**) exogenous contrast or pre–/post-processing required (0 = no; 1 = yes). After weighing the criterion, scores were summed to identify the most promising sequences for direct visualization of STN, GPi, and thalamic nuclei. Abbreviations: *DBS* deep brain stimulation, *FGATIR* fast gray matter acquisition T1w inversion recovery, *GP* globus pallidus, *QSM* quantitative susceptibility mapping, *STIR* short-T1 inversion recovery, *STN* subthalamic nucleus, *SWI* susceptibility-weighted imaging, *T* tesla, *Thal* thalamus, *WAIR* white matter attenuated inversion recovery

Most Common DBS Targets

Subthalamic Nucleus

The subthalamic nucleus (STN) is a small nucleus located inferior to the thalamus (Fig. 4.3). It is the most commonly used target for PD and has been trialed in the treatment of obsessive-compulsive disorder [8]. Anatomically, it is bounded by the internal capsule anterolaterally, the substantia nigra (SN) infero-laterally, cerebellothalamic fibers posteromedially, and fields of Forel and zona incerta superiorly [9]. Functionally, it is divided into a superior, posterior, and lateral sensorimotor area; a central associative area; and an emotive medial, anterior, and inferior tip [10].

Visualizing the STN

T2-weighted (T2w) and inversion recovery (IR) sequences remain the gold standard for DBS planning at most institutions. This reflects their ability to visualize the STN, but also their ease of implementation, widespread availability on most MRI

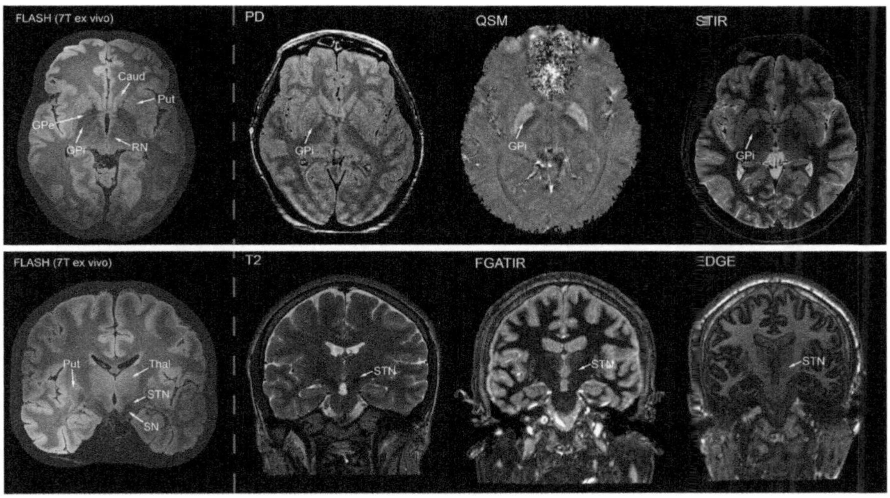

Fig. 4.3 Exemplar sequences for visualizing common DBS targets. First column: a high-resolution 7 T MRI [80] performed ex vivo clearly demonstrates STN and GPi, as well as neighboring anatomical structures. Top row: axial slices at the level of the pallidum are shown, demonstrating variable delineation of GPi. Bottom row: coronal slices at the level of the STN are shown, demonstrating variable separation of STN and neighboring SN. Abbreviations: *Caud* caudate, *EDGE* edge-enhancing gradient echo, *FGATIR* Fast Gray Matter Acquisition T1 Inversion Recovery, *GPi* globus pallidus internus, *GPe* globus pallidus externus, *FLASH* fast low angle shot, *PD* proton density, *Put* putamen, *QSM* quantitative susceptibility mapping, *RN* red nucleus, *STIR* short tau inversion recovery, *SN* substantia nigra, *STN* subthalamic nucleus, *T* tesla, *Thal* thalamus

vendor platforms, and accurate spatial representation of the structure [11]. As such, these are the sequences that novel techniques should be compared with. On T2w images, the STN is best appreciated on axial and coronal slices, and can be seen as a small—approximately 7 mm wide—hypointense structure [12–14]. The interface between the STN and SN is not always visible on T2w images, at 1.5 T [15] or 3 T [16]. Moreover, visualizing the STN on T2w sequences will only lead to improved targeting if stereotactic images are optimized for contrast and if they are processed to minimize distortion [17]. IR sequences aim to enhance the visualization of a given structure by selectively suppressing certain tissues with specific T1s. When using a fluid-attenuated inversion recovery (FLAIR) sequence, which nulls the signal from fluid, the STN remains hypointense with improved delineation compared to routine T2w imaging. Indeed, Senova et al. showed that preoperative targeting in PD patients at 3 T with a FLAIR sequence (3D SPACE [sampling perfection with application-optimized contrasts by using different flip angle evolution] FLAIR) was associated with both minimal geometric distortion and significantly higher contrast with surrounding structures, as well as better clinical outcomes at 12 months over routine T2w imaging [18]. However, similar to T2w sequences, the STN borders adjacent to the SN remain difficult to delineate, even at 3 T [12].

Other, less common IR sequences have also been used to visualize STN, such as short T1 inversion recovery (STIR), white matter attenuated Inversion recovery (WAIR), and fast gray matter T1 inversion recovery (FGATIR) [12, 19]. Notably, the STIR sequence has demonstrated increased contrast between the STN and SN at 3 T, offering improved delineation of the inferior STN border [20]. Recently, Zerroug et al. described their experience of using WAIR at 1.5 T for direct targeting in 156 patients, showing that the planned trajectory was chosen for implantation of definitive electrodes—optimized based on electrophysiological recording and awake stimulation testing—in 90.38% of cases [6]. Finally, FGATIR has shown promise in visualizing all STN borders in PD and ET patients, owing to increased contrast-to-noise ratio (CNR) [6, 21]. Despite promising results, such IR sequences are relatively underutilized in most centers. Their clinical performance against tried and trusted sequences should be assessed in larger, prospective studies.

SWI uses gradient echo (GRE) sequences to enhance the effect created by magnetic susceptibility differences between tissues. The paramagnetic property of iron—abundant within the STN—can be used to improve the STN's delineation from surrounding anatomy. SWI images, as well as accompanying T2*W [12, 22] and SWPI (susceptibility-weighted phase imaging) [23], have been successfully used to visualize all STN boundaries. In addition, Thaker et al. recently showed the use of a modified coronal GRE sequence to reliably visualize the neighboring rostral zona incerta in PD patients, which itself is a promising novel target for movement disorders [23, 24]. However, the biggest limitation of this technique is distortion—which has been shown to be >0.5 mm in x, y, and z planes when employing certain GRE sequences [25]—and overestimation of STN volume due to blooming artifacts. These distortions also render GRE sequences unusable for postoperative confirmation of electrode placement, in which there is considerable metal artifact.

To address some of the limitations of GRE sequences, post-processing techniques such as quantitative susceptibility mapping (QSM) have been developed to enable the quantification and mitigation of geometric distortions [16, 19]. QSM reduces the nonlocal susceptibility effect—which is the primary culprit in geometric distortions—by providing a clearer picture of tissue susceptibility and magnetic properties, regardless of patient and STN orientation [16, 26]. In addition, it provides a more accurate measurement of brain iron concentration, allowing for improved discrimination of surrounding iron-rich nuclei, such as the substantia nigra. Recently, Yu et al. showed the superiority of QSM—as measured by CNR and qualitative visualization scores—in delineating STN compared to a standard T2w sequence [27]. Rashid et al. also demonstrated the utility of this technique at 1.5 T by prospectively comparing direct targeting with QSM against a standard indirect targeting protocol. Across 11 patients, they showed that direct targeting with QSM resulted in statistically equivalent target coordinates compared to indirect targeting, highlighting opportunities for simpler and more intuitive surgical planning at centers with 1.5 T MRI [27, 28]. While the geometric accuracy of QSM post-processing has had limited clinical validation, Rasouli et al. showed a strong correlation of QSM with intraoperative microelectrode recording delineation of the STN in 25 PD patients [16]. Nonetheless, the technique lacks the simplicity with which standard T2 sequences can be acquired, and remains difficult to implement at many centers due to technical demands and complex offline post-processing [16, 29]. Based on a semi-quantitative evaluation of the literature, it appears susceptibility-based sequences and optimized IR sequences—including QSM, WAIR, and SWI 12, [12, 18, 20, 21, 30–35] may demonstrate superior target visibility compared with the more traditionally used T2w and IR (e.g., FLAIR) sequences (Table 4.2; Fig. 4.2). Further studies are necessary to validate the overall clinical performance and reliability of these less established sequences for preoperative planning.

Globus Pallidus

The GP is a lens-shaped gray matter structure situated between the putamen and internal capsule (Fig. 4.3). The putamen and GP are separated by the external medullary lamina, while the GP itself is subdivided by the medial medullary lamina into the globus pallidus internus (GPi) and externus (GPe) [21]. There is also an "accessary" medullary lamina within the GPi itself that partially subdivides it. GPi is bordered by the optic tract infero-medially and the internal capsule medially. The motor component is functionally segregated in the posterior GPi [36]. In clinical practice, the GPi is the second most common target for PD, and is the primary target for dystonia [36, 37].

Visualizing the GP

In our center's experience, proton density-weighted (PDW) sequences are most commonly used for direct visualization of the GP, which is best seen on axial and coronal slices [38, 39]. On T2w images, the GP can be seen as a hypointense structure [40], whereas it is slightly hyperintense on PDW images [39]. At lower field strengths (i.e., 1.5 T), these sequences generally visualize the optic tract, external medullary lamina and adjacent putamen, and the internal capsule bordering the posteromedial side of the GP. Optimized PD sequences are also readily able to delineate additional boundaries, such as the medial medullary lamina and accessory medial medullary lamina within the GPi [39]. Among other sequences, Nowacki et al. [41] investigated the use of a T1-weighted (T1w) sequence in dystonia patients, specifically the modified equilibrium Fourier transform (MDEFT) technique, which is employed at high field strengths due to its advantageous contrast characteristics. Using this MDEFT approach at 3 T field strength, the caudate putamen and pallidal subdivisions, the GPe and GPi, were well demarcated in most patients. Because the original surgical trajectory was used in patients undergoing microelectrode recording with multiple trajectories in 88% of all cases, MDEFT-based planning was deemed accurate and reliable.

IR sequences, on which the pallidum appears as a hypointense structure, have also been used. While IR spin echo sequences (e.g., IR-FSE) at 1.5 T have been shown to visualize the optic tract and external medullary lamina [40], FGATIR additionally allowed delineation of the internal medullary lamina [21, 40]. FGATIR has further been modified to enhance the distinction between the GPi and GPe by using parameters suppressing fluid and white matter (FLAWS) sequence [42]. In this study, FLAWS was generated through the registration of two contrasts, the standard T1-weighted anatomical contrast of the brain (i.e., magnetization-prepared rapid acquisition with gradient echo [MPRAGE]) and the suppression of the white matter signal (i.e., FGATIR), demonstrating enhanced visualization of subcortical structures in healthy participants.

As with the STN, susceptibility-based sequences permit direct visualization of the pallidum. T2*W and QSM sequences have been shown to discern the GPi and GPe in PD patients [27, 43]. However, with an SWI-like sequence at 3 T, Ide et al. [44] showed that the medial medullary lamina was less readily identifiable with increasing age, which may be related to increased mineralization in the GP and/or a loss of myelin.

Few studies have compared sequences for direct visualization of the GP and its subdivisions in a head-to-head manner. A handful of reports found that the GPi was best visualized using susceptibility-based sequences when compared with T1w, T2w, or IR sequences at 1.5 T and 3 T [32, 35, 38, 44]. Another found that, at 3 T, the internal medullary lamina in PD and ET patients was better visualized on an FGATIR sequence compared with the more commonly employed FLAIR and T1w imaging (i.e., MPRAGE) [21]. While these findings are not necessarily conflicting, additional studies comparing sequences would be helpful in establishing a consensus for optimal visualization of the pallidum and its internal architecture. Based on a semi-qualitative evaluation of the current literature, the most promising sequences for this purpose appear to be QSM, SWI, and FGATIR (Table 4.2; Fig. 4.2).

Table 4.2 Promising sequences for the direct visualization of common DBS targets

DSB target	Sequence	Designated as optimal by respective study	Described quality for direct visualization	Studied sample size	Scanned in disease population	Comparison with control subjects	Directly compared to other sequences within study	No post-processing required
STN	QSM Rasouli (2018)	1	3	3	1	1	1	0
STN	SWI Bus (2018)	1	3	3	1	0	2	1
STN	WAIR Zerroug (2016)	1	3	3	1	0	1	1
GPi	QSM Ide (2015)	1	3	3	1	1	1	0
GPi	FGATIR Sudhyadhom (2009)	1	3	1	1	0	2	1
GPi	SWI O'Gorman (2011)	1	2	3	0	0	2	1
Thal	FGATIR Morshita (2019)	1	3	1	1	0	1	1
Thal	WAIR Vassal (2012)	1	3	2	1	0	1	1
Thal	STIR Sarkar (2015)	1	3	3	0	1	1	1

For each target (i.e., STN, GP, or thalamus), studies performed using "clinical" (i.e., 1.5 T or 3 T MRI) field strengths were assessed and scored using a weighted decision matrix on nominal or ordinal scales. The top three sequences for each target according to this criterion are shown. The criterion included: (**a**) optimal sequence parameter from its respective study (0 = no; 1 = yes), (**b**) described quality when used for direct stereotactic targeting (1 = average; 2 = good; 3 = excellent), (**c**) sample size scanned (1 = 1–10; 2 = 11–20; 3 = ≥ 21 participants), (**d**) diseased populations scanned (0 = no; 1 = yes), (**e**) sequence was compared to controls (0 = no; 1 = yes), (**f**) number of sequences compared with (0 = none; 1 = 2–3; 2 = ≥ 4 sequences), and (**g**) exogenous contrast or pre–/post-processing required (1 = no; 0 = yes). After weighing the criterion, scores were summed to identify the most promising sequences for direct visualization of STN, GPi, and thalamic nuclei. According to these scores, the top three sequences for each target are shown. Abbreviations: *DBS* deep brain stimulation, *FGATIR* fast gray matter acquisition T1w inversion recovery, *GP* globus pallidus, *QSM* quantitative susceptibility mapping, *STIR* short-T1 inversion recovery, *STN* subthalamic nucleus, *SWI* susceptibility-weighted imaging, *T* tesla, *Thal* thalamus, *WAIR* white matter attenuated inversion recovery

Thalamus

The thalamus is superior to the hypothalamus and medial to the posterior limb of the internal capsule, forming the lateral wall of the third ventricle and floor of the lateral ventricles (Fig. 4.3). The thalamus is subdivided by the internal medullary lamina into anterior, mediodorsal, ventral, and lateral groups, with each group comprising several distinct nuclei [45]. Various thalamic nuclei have been targeted by DBS, including the ventral intermediate nucleus (Vim) (well-established in the treatment of tremor), ventrocaudal nucleus (for the management of chronic pain), centromedian nucleus (Tourette syndrome), and anterior nucleus of the thalamus (epilepsy) [37, 46].

Direct MRI Visualization

Thalamic nuclei are poorly appreciated on routine MRI sequences and often necessitate the use of atlas-derived coordinates for preoperative planning [37, 47]. On routinely acquired T1w and T2w sequences, the thalamus is mildly hyperintense and hypointense, respectively [37, 47, 48]. Despite its many nuclei, it appears fairly homogeneous with little distinction between subdivisions using standard parameters. However, studies in healthy participants have shown that the inversion time of T1w sequences may be optimized, allowing suppression of gray matter. The resulting gray and white matter differentiation enables identification of the main thalamic groups: anterior, dorsomedial, lateral, and ventral. Optimizing the repetition time of T1w (i.e., MPRAGE) has also been shown to enable specific delineation of the ANT, improving targeting prior to DBS epilepsy surgery [49]. To further optimize visualization of the thalamic nuclei, MPRAGE has been combined with phase data from 3D GRE sequences, which enabled the distinction of additional thalamic substructures such as the Vim [50]. Finally, multi-image co-registration and averaging of an MPRAGE sequence in healthy subjects has allowed delineation of the centromedian and parafascicular thalamic nuclei, which are promising targets for epilepsy and Tourette syndrome [50, 51]. While promising, these techniques have yet to be demonstrated in diseased populations and necessitate offline post-processing.

In one study using a 3 T PDW sequence, it was possible to visualize the Vim in healthy subjects as a mildly hypointense band crossing the anterior third of the thalamus, from lateral to medial [51, 52]. However, it was inconsistently seen at 1.5 T. Furthermore, the sensory thalamic nuclei (i.e., VC nucleus) were seen as another hypointense band located posteriorly [52]. Using PDW sequences at both 1.5 T and 3 T, two groups have reported direct targeting of the Vim in tremor patients [53, 54].

IR sequences have also enabled visualization of Vim. Specifically, studies have shown the Vim to be slightly hyperintense relative to the posterior nuclei on STIR sequences [55, 56]. IR sequences, including STIR and FGATIR, have also been used for targeting of the ANT based on delineation of the mammillothalamic tract, which terminates in ANT [48, 57, 58]. An IR sequence suppressing signal from white matter (i.e., white matter attenuated inversion recovery [WAIR]) has demonstrated significant enhancement of contrast between different gray matter territories in PD and ET patients, with promise in visualizing the internal subdivisions of the thalamus [59]. On WAIR, the Vim appears as a hypointense band crossing the ventrolateral region of the thalamus relative to the surrounding nuclei.

Across the very small number of studies comparing thalamic visualization sequences, IR sequences—specifically WAIR, STIR, and FGATIR—have been found to be superior to routinely used T1w imaging (Table 4.2; Fig. 4.2), while PDW sequences have been shown to be an improvement over T2w acquisitions [48, 53, 57].

Limitations

As highlighted in many of the aforementioned studies, advances in MRI sequences have allowed direct targeting to become more clinically feasible through improved visualization of subcortical structures [19]. However, there are common limitations evident within the existing literature that future studies may wish to address. Most apparently, there were few studies that directly and quantitatively compared sequences as to their ability to visualize DBS targets. Consequently, it is not possible to confidently conclude which sequences should be adopted for any given target. Further, additional studies are needed to determine whether direct targeting strategies are superior to indirect targeting in terms of clinical outcome, particularly when considering that the geometric distortions associated with many novel sequences have yet to be evaluated. Another caveat associated with certain studies was that images were acquired in healthy subjects rather than DBS patients, in whom target nuclei may be more difficult to appreciate [60, 61]. Finally, some sequences are limited by the need for using specific head coils that may not physically accommodate stereotactic head frames. While frameless techniques may be used, these may introduce errors inherent with MRI-CT or MRI-MRI co-registration that may further contribute to first-pass inaccuracy [62].

We attempted to systematically evaluate the utility of the sequences described in the literature for visualizing common DBS targets. However, this retrospective approach has several inherent limitations. While sequences were scored and ranked according to predefined criteria, it should be stressed that it is difficult to accurately compare sequences between studies. Further, the optimal sequences for each target may have been different if additional criteria were assessed, or if individual criteria were weighted differently. To truly establish the best sequences for direct visualization and preoperative planning, it is essential that future studies directly and objectively compare a priori chosen sequences in a prospective fashion according to clinically meaningful criteria.

Future Directions

The increasing availability of ultra-high field (UHF) MRI is likely to yield further improvements in the visualization of common DBS targets. Higher magnetic field strengths enable increased SNR and CNR, permitting increased spatial resolution and improving the ability to differentiate adjacent structures [63, 64]. It is not surprising then that UHF MRI has been shown to better visualize DBS targets—including STN and GPi [65]—than 1.5 T and 3 T [65, 66]. However, while higher magnetic field strengths may improve visualization, they are also more prone to susceptibility effects and image distortions [67], theoretically leading to a greater risk of mistargeting. That being said, higher field strengths also facilitate better acceleration factors and the development of advanced acquisitions which may be developed to mitigate these risks. Finally, while recent studies have shown preliminary evidence for the safety of DBS systems in UHF MRI, this has yet to be evaluated in vivo [68, 69].

Increasingly, there has been a shift in focus from what is being stimulated at the local level, toward what is being engaged at the network level [70]. Rather than discrete structures, such as deep gray matter nuclei, optimal targets may include white matter pathways [68, 71, 72] or focal hubs within larger functional networks [73]. To be appreciated, white matter tracts and functional networks require specialized MRI sequences, including diffusion MRI (dMRI) based tractography and functional magnetic resonance imaging (fMRI), respectively. Tractography-based targeting has already been used prospectively, with targeting of the dentato-rubro-thalamic tract (DRTT) and medial forebrain bundle for the treatment of essential tremor and psychiatric disorders, respectively [47, 74, 75]. Recently, probabilistic tractography has also been leveraged to provide reliable distinction of the motor and sensory thalamus for prospective targeting during asleep deep brain stimulation [76], and the protocol for a randomized controlled trial comparing the efficacy of the Vim-DBS (the traditional DBS target for tremor) and DRTT DBS has been published [77]. Beyond tractography, studies have hinted at the potential for using fMRI in operative planning. Notably, Younce et al. showed that preoperative resting-state functional connectivity (as assessed with resting state-fMRI) could predict clinical outcome, while Gibson et al. have shown that intraoperative fMRI can be used to determine engagement of distributed motor hubs associated with therapeutic effects [78, 79]. Overall, fMRI and tractography provide a potential opportunity to refine targeting using network-centered approaches (Fig. 4.4).

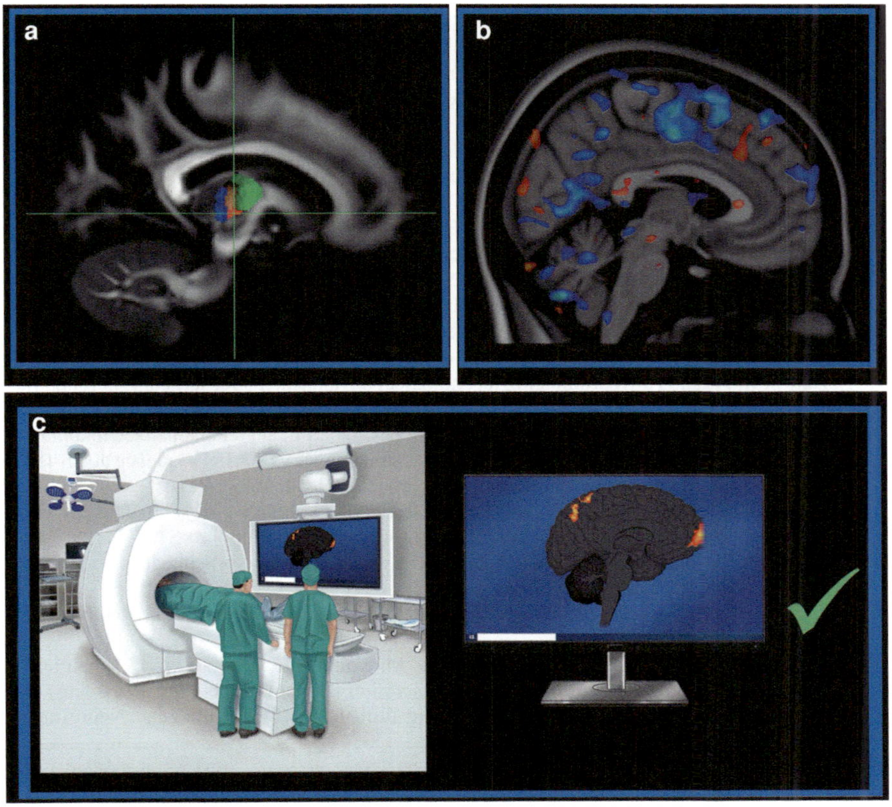

Fig. 4.4 Network-based approach to DBS target planning and lead insertion. MRI could be used to facilitate network-based target planning based on preoperative structural (**a**) and functional (**b**) connectivity. Panel A demonstrates parcellations of the thalamus based on structural connectivity to remote network hubs [47]. Intraoperative fMRI could be used to determine network engagement prior to final lead placement (**c**). Abbreviations: *DBS* deep brain stimulation, *fMRI* functional magnetic resonance imaging

Conclusions

Due to technological advances in neuroimaging, most DBS targets can currently be visualized on MRI to some degree, providing an adjunct or alternative to indirect targeting. Progress in this field largely stems from the development of optimized sequences and the increasing use of 3 T MRI in clinical settings, and it is expected that the visualization of DBS targets will only continue to improve. However, while direct targeting allows for anatomical variability between patients, encourages more individualized preoperative planning, and is more technically intuitive, studies are needed to objectively determine which visualization techniques are optimal for any given target.

References

1. Lemaire J-J, Coste J, Ouchchane L, et al. Brain mapping in stereotactic surgery: a brief overview from the probabilistic targeting to the patient-based anatomic mapping. NeuroImage. 2007;37(Suppl 1):S109–15.
2. Patel NK, Khan S, Gill SS. Comparison of atlas- and magnetic-resonance-imaging-based stereotactic targeting of the subthalamic nucleus in the surgical treatment of Parkinson's disease. Stereotact Funct Neurosurg. 2008;86:153–61.
3. Bejjani BP, Dormont D, Pidoux B, et al. Bilateral subthalamic stimulation for Parkinson's disease by using three-dimensional stereotactic magnetic resonance imaging and electrophysiological guidance. J Neurosurg. 2000;92:615–25.
4. Zrinzo L, Hariz M, Hyam JA, Foltynie T, Limousin P. Letter to the editor: a paradigm shift toward MRI-guided and MRI-verified DBS surgery. J Neurosurg. 2016;124:1135–7.
5. Boutet A, Gramer R, Steele CJ, Elias GJB, Germann J, Maciel R, Kucharczyk W, Zrinzo L, Lozano AM, Fasano A. Neuroimaging technological advancements for targeting in functional neurosurgery. Curr Neurol Neurosci Rep. 2019;19:42.
6. Zerroug A, Gabrillargues J, Coll G, Vassal F, Jean B, Chabert E, et al. Personalized mapping of the deep brain with a white matter attenuated inversion recovery (WAIR) sequence at 1.5-tesla: experience based on a series of 156 patients. Neurochirurgie. 2016;62:183–9.
7. Benabid AL, Koudsie A, Benazzouz A, Le Bas J-F, Pollak P. Imaging of subthalamic nucleus and ventralis intermedius of the thalamus. Mov Disord. 2002;17(Suppl 3):S123–9.
8. Lozano AM, Lipsman N. Probing and regulating dysfunctional circuits using deep brain stimulation. Neuron. 2013;77:406–24.
9. Weintraub DB, Zaghloul KA. The role of the subthalamic nucleus in cognition. Rev Neurosci. 2013;24:125–38.
10. Lambert C, Zrinzo L, Nagy Z, Lutti A, Hariz M, Foltynie T, Draganski B, Ashburner J, Frackowiak R. Confirmation of functional zones within the human subthalamic nucleus: patterns of connectivity and sub-parcellation using diffusion weighted imaging. NeuroImage. 2012;60:83–94.
11. Brunenberg EJL, Platel B, Hofman PAM, ter Haar Romeny BM, Visser-Vandewalle V. Magnetic resonance imaging techniques for visualization of the subthalamic nucleus. J Neurosurg. 2011;115:971–84.
12. Kerl HU, Gerigk L, Pechlivanis I, Al-Zghloul M, Groden C, Nölte I. The subthalamic nucleus at 3.0 tesla: choice of optimal sequence and orientation for deep brain stimulation using a standard installation protocol: clinical article. J Neurosurg. 2012;117:1155–65.
13. Dormont D, Ricciardi KG, Tandé D, Parain K, Menuel C, Galanaud D, Navarro S, Cornu P, Agid Y, Yelnik J. Is the subthalamic nucleus hypointense on T2-weighted images? A correlation study using MR imaging and stereotactic atlas data. AJNR Am J Neuroradiol. 2004;25:1516–23.
14. Mai JK, Majtanik M, Paxinos G. Atlas of the human brain. Academic Press; 2015.
15. Danish SF, Jaggi JL, Moyer JT, Finkel L, Baltuch GH. Conventional MRI is inadequate to delineate the relationship between the red nucleus and subthalamic nucleus in Parkinson's disease. Stereotact Funct Neurosurg. 2006;84:12–8.
16. Rasouli J, Ramdhani R, Panov FE, Dimov A, Zhang Y, Cho C, Wang Y, Kopell BH. Utilization of quantitative susceptibility mapping for direct targeting of the subthalamic nucleus during deep brain stimulation surgery. Oper Neurosurg (Hagerstown). 2018;14:412–9.
17. Zonenshayn M, Rezai AR, Mogilner AY, Beric A, Sterio D, Kelly PJ. Comparison of anatomic and neurophysiological methods for subthalamic nucleus targeting. Neurosurgery. 2000;47(282–92):discussion 292–4.
18. Senova S, Hosomi K, Gurruchaga J-M, et al. Three-dimensional SPACE fluid-attenuated inversion recovery at 3 T to improve subthalamic nucleus lead placement for deep brain stimulation in Parkinson's disease: from preclinical to clinical studies. J Neurosurg. 2016;125:472–80.
19. Chandran AS, Bynevelt M, Lind CRP. Magnetic resonance imaging of the subthalamic nucleus for deep brain stimulation. J Neurosurg. 2016;124:96–105.

20. Kitajima M, Korogi Y, Kakeda S, Moriya J, Ohnari N, Sato T, Hayashida Y, Hirai T, Okuda T, Yamashita Y. Human subthalamic nucleus: evaluation with high-resolution MR imaging at 3.0 T. Neuroradiology. 2008;50:675–81.
21. Sudhyadhom A, Haq IU, Foote KD, Okun MS, Bova FJ. A high resolution and high contrast MRI for differentiation of subcortical structures for DBS targeting: the fast gray matter acquisition T1 inversion recovery (FGATIR). NeuroImage. 2009;47(Suppl 2):T44–52.
22. Xiao Y, Fonov V, Bériault S, Al Subaie F, Chakravarty MM, Sadikot AF, Pike GB, Collins DL. Multi-contrast unbiased MRI atlas of a Parkinson's disease population. Int J Comput Assist Radiol Surg. 2015;10:329–41.
23. Vertinsky AT, Coenen VA, Lang DJ, Kolind S, Honey CR, Li D, Rauscher A. Localization of the subthalamic nucleus: optimization with susceptibility-weighted phase MR imaging. AJNR Am J Neuroradiol. 2009;30:1717–24.
24. Thaker AA, Reddy KM, Thompson JA, Gerecht PD, Brown MS, Abosch A, Ojemann SG, Kern DS. Coronal gradient Echo MRI to visualize the zona Incerta for deep brain stimulation targeting in Parkinson's disease. SFN. 2021;99:443–50.
25. Watanabe Y, Lee CK, Gerbi BJ. Geometrical accuracy of a 3-tesla magnetic resonance imaging unit in gamma knife surgery. J Neurosurg. 2006;105:190–3.
26. Li J, Chang S, Liu T, et al. Reducing the object orientation dependence of susceptibility effects in gradient echo MRI through quantitative susceptibility mapping. Magn Reson Med. 2012;68:1563–9.
27. Yu K, Ren Z, Li J, Guo S, Hu Y, Li Y. Direct visualization of deep brain stimulation targets in patients with Parkinson's disease via 3-T quantitative susceptibility mapping. Acta Neurochir. 2021;163:1335–45.
28. Rashid T, Hwang R, DiMarzio M, Hancu I, Pilitsis JG. Evaluating the role of 1.5 T quantitative susceptibility mapping for subthalamic nucleus targeting in deep brain stimulation surgery. J Neuroradiol. 2021;48:37–42.
29. Schweser F, Deistung A, Reichenbach JR. Foundations of MRI phase imaging and processing for quantitative susceptibility mapping (QSM). Z Med Phys. 2016;26:6–34.
30. Heo YJ, Kim SJ, Kim HS, Choi CG, Jung SC, Lee JK, Lee CS, Chung SJ, Cho SH, Lee GR. Three-dimensional fluid-attenuated inversion recovery sequence for visualisation of subthalamic nucleus for deep brain stimulation in Parkinson's disease. Neuroradiology. 2015;57:929–35.
31. Ben-Haim S, Gologorsky Y, Monahan A, Weisz D, Alterman RL. Fiducial registration with spoiled gradient-echo magnetic resonance imaging enhances the accuracy of subthalamic nucleus targeting. Neurosurgery. 2011;69:870–5. discussion 875.
32. Liu T, Eskreis-Winkler S, Schweitzer AD, Chen W, Kaplitt MG, Tsiouris AJ, Wang Y. Improved subthalamic nucleus depiction with quantitative susceptibility mapping. Radiology. 2013;269:216–23.
33. Lefranc M, Derrey S, Merle P, et al. High-resolution 3-dimensional T2*-weighted angiography (HR 3-D SWAN): an optimized 3-T magnetic resonance imaging sequence for targeting the subthalamic nucleus. Neurosurgery. 2014;74:615–26. discussion 627.
34. Nagahama H, Suzuki K, Shonai T, Aratani K, Sakurai Y, Nakamura M, Sakata M. Comparison of magnetic resonance imaging sequences for depicting the subthalamic nucleus for deep brain stimulation. Radiol Phys Technol. 2015;8:30–5.
35. O'Gorman RL, Shmueli K, Ashkan K, Samuel M, Lythgoe DJ, Shahidiani A, Wastling SJ, Footman M, Selway RP, Jarosz J. Optimal MRI methods for direct stereotactic targeting of the subthalamic nucleus and globus pallidus. Eur Radiol. 2011;21:130–6.
36. Ewert S, Plettig P, Li N, Chakravarty MM, Collins DL, Herrington TM, Kühn AA, Horn A. Toward defining deep brain stimulation targets in MNI space: a subcortical atlas based on multimodal MRI, histology and structural connectivity. NeuroImage. 2018;170:271–82.
37. Lozano AM, Lipsman N, Bergman H, et al. Deep brain stimulation: current challenges and future directions. Nat Rev Neurol. 2019;15:148–60.
38. Nölte IS, Gerigk L, Al-Zghloul M, Groden C, Kerl HU. Visualization of the internal globus pallidus: sequence and orientation for deep brain stimulation using a standard installation protocol at 3.0 tesla. Acta Neurochir. 2012;154:481–94.

39. Hirabayashi H, Tengvar M, Hariz MI. Stereotactic imaging of the pallidal target. Mov Disord. 2002;17(Suppl 3):S130–4.
40. Starr PA, Vitek JL, DeLong M, Bakay RA. Magnetic resonance imaging-based stereotactic localization of the globus pallidus and subthalamic nucleus. Neurosurgery. 1999;44:303–13. discussion 313–4.
41. Nowacki A, Fiechter M, Fichtner J, Debove I, Lachenmayer L, Schüpbach M, Oertel MF, Wiest R, Pollo C. Using MDEFT MRI sequences to target the GPi in DBS surgery. PLoS One. 2015;10:e0137868.
42. Beaumont J, Saint-Jalmes H, Acosta O, Kober T, Tanner M, Ferré JC, Salvado O, Fripp J, Gambarota G. Multi T1-weighted contrast MRI with fluid and white matter suppression at 1.5 T. Magn Reson Imaging. 2019;63:217–25.
43. Ide S, Kakeda S, Ueda I, et al. Internal structures of the globus pallidus in patients with Parkinson's disease: evaluation with quantitative susceptibility mapping (QSM). Eur Radiol. 2015;25:710–8.
44. Ide S, Kakeda S, Yoneda T, et al. Internal structures of the Globus pallidus in patients with Parkinson's disease: evaluation with phase difference-enhanced imaging. Magn Reson Med Sci. 2017;16:304–10.
45. Nieuwenhuys R, Voogd J, van Huijzen C. The human central nervous system: a synopsis and atlas. Springer Science & Business Media; 2013.
46. Hamani C, Schwalb JM, Rezai AR, Dostrovsky JO, Davis KD, Lozano AM. Deep brain stimulation for chronic neuropathic pain: long-term outcome and the incidence of insertional effect. Pain. 2006;125:188–96.
47. Akram H, Dayal V, Mahlknecht P, et al. Connectivity derived thalamic segmentation in deep brain stimulation for tremor. Neuroimage Clin. 2018;18:130–42.
48. Grewal SS, Middlebrooks EH, Kaufmann TJ, Stead M, Lundstrom BN, Worrell GA, Lin C, Baydin S, Van Gompel JJ. Fast gray matter acquisition T1 inversion recovery MRI to delineate the mammillothalamic tract for preoperative direct targeting of the anterior nucleus of the thalamus for deep brain stimulation in epilepsy. Neurosurg Focus. 2018;45:E6.
49. Buentjen L, Kopitzki K, Schmitt FC, Voges J, Tempelmann C, Kaufmann J, Kanowski M. Direct targeting of the thalamic anteroventral nucleus for deep brain stimulation by T1-weighted magnetic resonance imaging at 3 T. Stereotact Funct Neurosurg. 2014;92:25–30.
50. Bender B, Wagner S, Klose U. Optimized depiction of thalamic substructures with a combination of T1-MPRAGE and phase: MPRAGE. Clin Neuroradiol. 2017;27:511–8.
51. Middlebrooks EH, Okromelidze L, Lin C, Jain A, Westerhold E, Ritaccio A, Quiñones-Hinojosa A, Gupta V, Grewal SS. Edge-enhancing gradient echo with multi-image co-registration and averaging (EDGE-MICRA) for targeting thalamic centromedian and parafascicular nuclei. Neuroradiol J. 2021;19714009211021781
52. Spiegelmann R, Nissim O, Daniels D, Ocherashvilli A, Mardor Y. Stereotactic targeting of the ventrointermediate nucleus of the thalamus by direct visualization with high-field MRI. Stereotact Funct Neurosurg. 2006;84:19–23.
53. Morrison MA, Lee AT, Martin AJ, Dietiker C, Brown EG, Wang DD. DBS targeting for essential tremor using intersectional dentato-rubro-thalamic tractography and direct proton density visualization of the VIM: technical note on 2 cases. J Neurosurg. 2021;135:806–14.
54. Sidiropoulos C, Mubita L, Krstevska S, Schwalb JM. Successful vim targeting for mixed essential and parkinsonian tremor using intraoperative MRI. J Neurol Sci. 2015;358:488–9.
55. Alterman RL, Reiter GT, Shils J, Skolnick B, Arle JE, Lesutis M, Simuni T, Colcher A, Stern M, Hurtig H. Targeting for thalamic deep brain stimulator implantation without computer guidance: assessment of targeting accuracy. Stereotact Funct Neurosurg. 1999;72:150–3.
56. Yamada K, Akazawa K, Yuen S, Goto M, Matsushima S, Takahata A, Nakagawa M, Mineura K, Nishimura T. MR imaging of ventral thalamic nuclei. AJNR Am J Neuroradiol. 2010;31:732–5.
57. Jiltsova E, Möttönen T, Fahlström M, Haapasalo J, Tähtinen T, Peltola J, Öhman J, Larsson E-M, Kiekara T, Lehtimäki K. Imaging of anterior nucleus of thalamus using 1.5T MRI for deep brain stimulation targeting in refractory epilepsy. Neuromodulation. 2016;19:812–7.

58. Möttönen T, Katisko J, Haapasalo J, Tähtinen T, Kiekara T, Kähärä V, Peltola J, Öhman J, Lehtimäki K. Defining the anterior nucleus of the thalamus (ANT) as a deep brain stimulation target in refractory epilepsy: delineation using 3 T MRI and intraoperative microelectrode recording. Neuroimage Clin. 2015;7:823–9.
59. Vassal F, Coste J, Derost P, Mendes V, Gabrillargues J, Nuti C, Durif F, Lemaire J-J. Direct stereotactic targeting of the ventrointermediate nucleus of the thalamus based on anatomic 1.5-T MRI mapping with a white matter attenuated inversion recovery (WAIR) sequence. Brain Stimul. 2012;5:625–33.
60. Bonneville F, Welter ML, Elie C, et al. Parkinson disease, brain volumes, and subthalamic nucleus stimulation. Neurology. 2005;64:1598–604.
61. Lee SH, Kim SS, Tae WS, Lee SY, Choi JW, Koh SB, Kwon DY. Regional volume analysis of the Parkinson disease brain in early disease stage: gray matter, white matter, striatum, and thalamus. AJNR Am J Neuroradiol. 2011;32:682–7.
62. O'Gorman RL, Jarosz JM, Samuel M, Clough C, Selway RP, Ashkan K. CT/MR image fusion in the postoperative assessment of electrodes implanted for deep brain stimulation. Stereotact Funct Neurosurg. 2009;87:205–10.
63. Kraff O, Quick HH. 7T: physics, safety, and potential clinical applications. J Magn Reson Imaging. 2017;46:1573–89.
64. Springer E, Dymerska B, Cardoso PL, Robinson SD, Weisstanner C, Wiest R, Schmitt B, Trattnig S. Comparison of routine brain imaging at 3 T and 7 T. Investig Radiol. 2016;51:469–82.
65. Cong F, Liu X, Liu C-SJ, Xu X, Shen Y, Wang B, Zhuo Y, Yan L. Improved depiction of subthalamic nucleus and globus pallidus internus with optimized high-resolution quantitative susceptibility mapping at 7 T. NMR Biomed. 2020;33:e4382.
66. Abosch A, Yacoub E, Ugurbil K, Harel N. An assessment of current brain targets for deep brain stimulation surgery with susceptibility-weighted imaging at 7 tesla. Neurosurgery. 2010;67:1745–56. discussion 1756.
67. Dammann P, Kraff O, Wrede KH, et al. Evaluation of hardware-related geometrical distortion in structural MRI at 7 tesla for image-guided applications in neurosurgery. Acad Radiol. 2011;18:910–6.
68. Hoff MN, McKinney A 4th, Shellock FG, Rassner U, Gilk T, Watson RE Jr, Greenberg TD, Froelich J, Kanal E. Safety considerations of 7-T MRI in clinical practice. Radiology. 2019;292:509–18.
69. Bhusal B, Stockmann J, Guerin B, et al. Safety and image quality at 7T MRI for deep brain stimulation systems: ex vivo study with lead-only and full-systems. PLoS One. 2021;16:e0257077.
70. Horn A, Fox MD. Opportunities of connectomic neuromodulation. NeuroImage. 2020;221:117180.
71. Yarach U, Luengviriya C, Stucht D, Godenschweger F, Schulze P, Speck O. Correction of B 0-induced geometric distortion variations in prospective motion correction for 7T MRI. MAGMA. 2016;29:319–32.
72. See AAQ, King NKK. Improving surgical outcome using diffusion tensor imaging techniques in deep brain stimulation. Front Surg. 2017;4:54.
73. Horn A, Reich M, Vorwerk J, et al. Connectivity predicts deep brain stimulation outcome in Parkinson disease. Ann Neurol. 2017;82:67–78.
74. Coenen VA, Allert N, Paus S, Kronenbürger M, Urbach H, Mädler B. Modulation of the cerebello-thalamo-cortical network in thalamic deep brain stimulation for tremor: a diffusion tensor imaging study. Neurosurgery. 2014;75:657–69. discussion 669–70.
75. Coenen VA, Sajonz B, Reisert M, Bostroem J, Bewernick B, Urbach H, Jenkner C, Reinacher PC, Schlaepfer TE, Mädler B. Tractography-assisted deep brain stimulation of the superolateral branch of the medial forebrain bundle (slMFB DBS) in major depression. Neuroimage Clin. 2018;20:580–93.
76. Muller J, Alizadeh M, Matias CM, Thalheimer S, Romo V, Martello J, Liang T-W, Mohamed FB, Wu C. Use of probabilistic tractography to provide reliable distinction of the motor and sensory thalamus for prospective targeting during asleep deep brain stimulation. J Neurosurg. 2021:1–10.

77. Sajonz BEA, Amtage F, Reinacher PC, Jenkner C, Piroth T, Kätzler J, Urbach H, Coenen VA. Deep brain stimulation for tremor Tractographic versus traditional (DISTINCT): study protocol of a randomized controlled feasibility trial. JMIR Res Protoc. 2016;5:e244.
78. Gibson WS, Jo HJ, Testini P, Cho S, Felmlee JP, Welker KM, Klassen BT, Min H-K, Lee KH. Functional correlates of the therapeutic and adverse effects evoked by thalamic stimulation for essential tremor. Brain. 2016;139:2198–210.
79. Younce JR, Campbell MC, Hershey T, et al. Resting-state functional connectivity predicts STN DBS clinical response. Mov Disord. 2021;36:662–71.
80. Edlow BL, Mareyam A, Horn A, et al (2019) 7 tesla MRI of the ex vivo human brain at 100 micron resolution. Sci Data. 2019; https://doi.org/10.1038/s41597-019-0254-8.

Safety of Magnetic Resonance Imaging in Patients with Deep Brain Stimulation

5

Clement T. Chow, Sriranga Kashyap, Aaron Loh, Asma Naheed, Nicole Bennett, Laleh Golestanirad, and Alexandre Boutet

Introduction

Magnetic resonance imaging (MRI) provides invaluable information to clinicians and researchers that other imaging modalities such as computed tomography scan cannot provide. New comorbidities that arise in patients following DBS surgery, such as cerebrovascular disease, require MRI but only 5% of patients with DBS devices in whom MRI is indicated are actually scanned [1]. Each institution's MR

C. T. Chow (✉)
University Health Network, Toronto, ON, Canada

Division of Neurosurgery, Toronto Western Hospital, Toronto, ON, Canada
e-mail: clem.chow@mail.utoronto.ca

S. Kashyap · A. Loh
University Health Network, Toronto, ON, Canada
e-mail: Sriranga.Kashyap@rmp.uhn.ca; aaron.loh@mail.utoronto.ca

A. Naheed · N. Bennett
Joint Department of Medical Imaging, University of Toronto, Toronto, ON, Canada
e-mail: Asma.Naheed@uhn.ca; Nicole.Bennett@uhn.ca

L. Golestanirad
Department of Radiology, Feinberg School of Medicine, Northwestern University, Chicago, IL, USA

Department of Biomedical Engineering, McCormick School of Engineering, Northwestern University, Evanston, IL, USA
e-mail: laleh.rad1@northwestern.edu

A. Boutet
University Health Network, Toronto, ON, Canada

Joint Department of Medical Imaging, University of Toronto, Toronto, ON, Canada
e-mail: alexandre.boutet@mail.utoronto.ca

A. Boutet, A. M. Lozano (eds.), *Magnetic Resonance Imaging in Deep Brain Stimulation*, https://doi.org/10.1007/978-3-031-16348-7_5

safety policies regarding scanning DBS devices are site-specific and usually significantly restrictive.

DBS devices are considered active implantable medical devices (AIMDs) and some are classified as MR Conditional (i.e., patients with this device or object may be scanned safely but are subject to compliance with certain specified conditions) [2, 3]. AIMDs are powered through a built-in battery or internal pulse generator (e.g., DBS Medtronic Percept PC), or through a coupled external supply (e.g., DBS Medtronic SE-4). These are at an additional risk of malfunction, modification in their operation mode, inhibition, unintended stimulation, and/or permanent damage to the unit [4].

Given the history of MR-related injuries in patients with DBS devices, preventative measures are taken by precluding patients with devices or implants that might create a health risk or interfere with the MRI [5]. The possibility for MR-induced device heating generated by radiofrequency (RF) exposure, amongst other risks, could lead to detrimental brain damage [6–8]. Neural tissues are extremely sensitive to even modest temperature elevations and permanent brain damage can occur at 45 °C (i.e., 7–8 °C in excess of normal body temperature). Although there are no guidelines ascertaining a safe limit of RF heating of the brain tissue, temperature increases below 2 °C have been deemed to be safe as this temperature elevation is comparable to a low-grade fever [9].

In this chapter, we discuss: (1) the standard method of safety testing and the importance of emulating device configuration and positioning, (2) the unpredictable nature of MR-induced heating, (3) the findings from MR safety studies performed in humans, (4) special considerations when operating with high-field MR units or performing advanced sequence parameters, and (5) innovations, tools, and policies designed to safeguard against MR hazards.

Standards of Safety Testing

Magnetic Field Components within the Suite

The MR environment is composed of three magnetic fields: 1) the main static field (B_0), 2) the RF pulses (B_1), and 3) the gradients (dB/dt) responsible for spatial localization [10]. Each of these raise different safety concerns for DBS patients (summarized in Table 5.1). Each safety concern has a designated standard guidelines for safety testing set forth by the American Society for Testing and Materials (ASTM) [9, 11, 12] or International Organization for Standardization Technical Standard (ISO/TS), [13] and incorporated into the standards of the International Electrotechnical Commission (IEC) [14]. ASTM testing standards require the use of phantom models which are standardized containers commonly filled with a semi-solid gel containing a polyacrylic acid or saline medium designed to simulate thermal and electrical properties of neural tissues (see Fig. 5.1) [9, 11–13]. The following

Table 5.1 Safety concerns contributed by each component of the MR environment

Components of MR environment	Physical MR-induced effects	Potential adverse effects to patient	Testing standard	Acceptance criterion
Static Magnetic Field—Always present	Rotational force (torque) on electrodes, IPG	Tearing of tissues; rotation of DBS components to align with field	ASTM F2213-17, low friction surface method	Torque less than gravitational torque
Static Magnetic Field Spatial Gradient—Always present	Translational force on electrodes, IPG	Tearing of tissues; acceleration of implant; "missile effect"	ASTM F2052-15	Magnetic force less than medical device weight
	Lenz force from rapid motion in a direction perpendicular to B_0 orientation	Tugging or pulling on implant with excessive movement		
Gradient Magnetic Field—Pulsed during imaging	Induced currents in DBS extensions/electrode due to dB/dt	Device malfunction or failure of DBS-ON	Device interrogation following scan	No device malfunction, interference, altered settings or permanent damage.
Radio frequency Field—Pulsed during imaging	RF-induced currents resulting in electrode heating of tissue	Overheating of tissues; thermal and electrical burns; antenna effect	ASTM F2182-19e2	Change in heating less than 2 °C
	Electromagnetic interference of DBS-ON	Device malfunctioning; induced noise	Device interrogation following scan	No device malfunction, interference, altered settings or permanent damage

three sections will discuss theoretical safety risks and findings from phantoms (findings from human studies will be presented separately).

Heterogeneity in Implanted Configurations and Positioning

When conducting site-specific, "local" testing with phantom models, the DBS configuration should emulate the institution-specific implantation arrangement in terms of electrode quantity (bilateral versus unilateral implants), placement of excess extension wires, and internal pulse generator (IPG) positioning. Several studies have reported rises in temperature on the contralateral electrode to the IPG compared to the ipsilateral electrode [15], or the excess coiling behind the IPG, found in

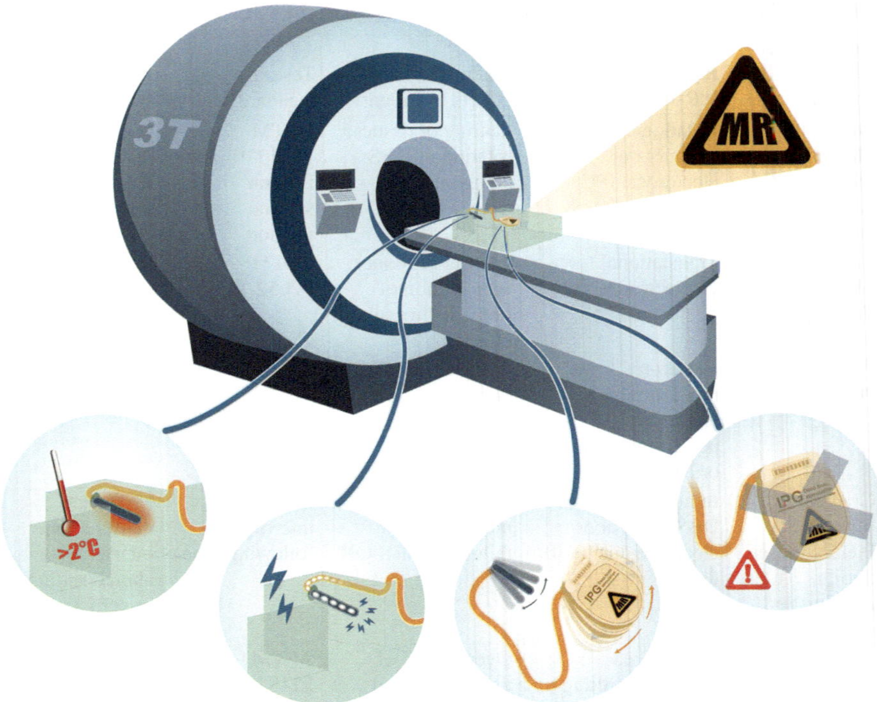

Fig. 5.1 Phantom filled with a semisolid polyacrylamide gel used to test the main hazards of performing magnetic resonance imaging with a deep brain stimulation device. (From left to right) (i) heating at the electrode tips, (ii) unintended stimulation, (iii) translation displacement, torque, or vibrations of device components, (iv) device integrity is compromised or malfunctioning

the thoracic area, may lead to marked temperature rises as opposed to subgaleal coiling in the head area [16, 17]. Unilateral and bilateral IPG configurations also influence heating differently with the latter increasing temperatures more than the former configuration [18]. Furthermore, older MRI safety studies are configured in a way where the testing simulates the "first stage" of staged DBS surgeries when systems are not considered fully implanted. In particular, the first stage only comprises electrodes implanted in the target structure with the extracranial portion of the lead routed under the scalp. In the second stage, fully-implanted systems have leads connected to extensions, which are then routed subcutaneously down the neck and connected to the IPG in the infraclavicular region [19]. Thus, it is important to consider the configuration and position of the device in the RF and gradient fields relative to the MR coil when scanning patients. Other than the physical configurations of the DBS device and positioning of the patient within the MR bore, (1) heating at the electrode tips, (2) induced currents, (3) mechanical forces, and (4) implantable pulse generator dysfunction must also be accounted for (these factors will be discussed in the following sections).

MR-Induced Heating Concerns

The Unpredictable Nature of Heating

Heating caused by the RF pulses is termed "resonant heating" (also known as the antenna effect). Resonant heating primarily occurs when the length of the DBS leads or extensions are approximately half the wavelength of emitted RF pulses. MRI at different field strengths emit RF pulses at different resonant (Larmor) frequencies for ^{1}H nuclei (64 MHz at 1.5 T and 127 MHz at 3 T MRI) which can be intercepted by conductive DBS components approximately 29 cm long in 1.5 T or 15 cm long in 3 T MRI analogous to a common wire antenna (hence the "antenna effect") [20]. However, there is an extra degree of complexity as the resonant wavelengths vary considerably from tissue to tissue since the wavelength is dependent on the unique dielectric properties (i.e., permittivity) of the tissue type. Furthermore, the physical length of the implanted lead may not reflect the true length or design of the conductive material within (i.e., there may be internal loops or redundancy of conductive elements within the lead), making resonant conditions arise unpredictably from leads of a variety of physical lengths. The degree of heating can reach >10 °C within seconds early in an acquisition at the tips of the electrodes, but other complex interactions within the MR environment can also contribute to heating [10].

Heating unpredictably varies across scanners, devices, imaging techniques, electromagnetic interference, human factors, position within the fields amongst other factors. Heating can result from RF pulses emitted at tissues or resonant heating. Although for the same generated images, a 3 T scanner will produce more heating than a 1.5 T scanner. The scenario can dramatically change in the presence of elongated leads due to the resonance effect. In fact, components within the DBS device could theoretically be more susceptible to resonant heating at 1.5 T rather than 3 T due to their dimensions. Studies conducting physical safety experiments have found that temperature rises between 1.5 and 3 T were not significantly different (< 1° increase difference) [21, 22]. In other words, risk assessments are not straightforward and immediate specifications of an MRI scanner (e.g., field strength) should not predetermine whether a patient is scanned. Rather, vendor guidelines to SAR and B_{1+rms} limits of a particular device should always be followed to determine safety. For example, two systems of different generations—but the same vendor, field strength, similar coils, and RF power deposition—resulted in a significant difference in averaged body SAR (albeit sequence parameters were not provided and gradients between the scanners were different) [23, 24]. Different coils (body-transmit versus head-transmit), clinical and research pulse sequences employing varying levels of RF energy, and phantoms containing different concentrations of polyacrylic acid may also result in inconsistent temperature rises [17]. Thus, results from past studies are usually difficult to replicate because of variations in the MRI hardware and software, DBS systems, and testing materials.

Measuring Heating

With the DBS leads implanted in thermally brain sensitive tissues, it is essential that assessment of conditions for safe scanning are made with the DBS device in its entirety, after identifying all implanted components of the system. Limiting the assessment only to those related, for example, to the IPG (typically implanted in the thoracic region), without appreciating conditions associated with the leads tunneled subcutaneously towards the burr holes, or electrodes implanted into designated anatomic targets could pose significant patient hazards.

When testing in phantoms, temperature recordings are measured with a thermometry probe at the location suspected of having the highest increases in heating and/or locations of tissues most sensitive to temperature changes. In the case of DBS devices, this is typically at the tips of the electrodes where stimulation of brain structures occurs [9, 11, 12]. FDA guidelines use specific absorption rate (SAR), a conservative RF exposure estimate of energy deposited in a region (e.g., head, whole-body, partial body) during a pulse sequence [3, 23, 24]. Each DBS vendor has recommended SAR limits for each product and these recommendations are more restrictive than the FDA's general SAR requirements for humans undergoing MRI.

Alternatively, the B_1^+ field root-mean-square (B_{1+rms}) is a time-averaged value of the effective transmit (+) component of the B_1 field strength employed during MR image creation [25]. DBS vendor guidelines recommend that scanning should not exceed the recommended SAR or B_{1+rms} limits for particular DBS models. Using B_{1+rms} may resolve some of the inherent limitations of SAR, but is far from being an ideal measure of heating [26]. Predicting SAR is dependent on factors such as the known B_{1+rms} value, morphology, tissue composition, posture, landmark location, and averaging time. Conversely, B_{1+rms}—which is less restrictive within the DBS vendor guidelines—is a fundamental electromagnetic field parameter more dependent on the incident RF field rather than the patient's absorption of RF within the body.

Other Potential MRI-Related Risks

Unintended Stimulation

The electrode tip is the location where the electrical current flux density is highest in resonant conditions, as well as the location with the highest resistance. This can possibly induce unintended stimulation, depending on the position of the electrodes in the brain and exposure to the RF or gradient fields [20]. Induced voltages of up to 1.5 V have been recorded in studies investigating the IPG output during 1.5 T and 3 T MRI [22]. However, induced voltages should not be of clinical concern since IPGs typically stimulate at 3 to 6 V in clinical practice for Parkinson's disease patients [21, 27]. Additional low voltages induced by the RF pulses or applied gradient field superimposed on the stimulation of the DBS system and discomfort experienced by patients are seldom reported [22, 28, 29].

Magnetically Induced Displacement or Vibrations

Modern day neurostimulators are non-magnetic or diamagnetic, and strong magnetically induced rotational and translational forces (known as the "missile effect") are not expected [28, 30]. However, vibrations induced by eddy currents on the conductive surfaces of DBS components can theoretically lead to breakage of internal components and subsequently device malfunctioning. Consistent with the fact that DBS systems have demonstrated to be non-ferrous in nature, the risk of implant motion tends to be trivial for smaller implanted leads or electrodes [31]. More recent studies have shown that Medtronic Activa PC devices do not generate any gross translation or torque forces on the IPG [21, 22, 26]. Obsolete DBS devices with RF receivers and a separate RF transmitter (i.e., Medtronic Itrel II) may contain residual magnetic materials, such as sealing chips, ferrite core antennas, and reed switches that might move or dislodge the device from its implanted position [30]. For this, older studies testing dated DBS models may not be relevant to current DBS devices (i.e., Medtronic Percept PC is full-body MR Conditional at 1.5 and 3 T) [16, 17, 23, 28, 30, 32–38]. Further, the majority of studies in the literature examine Medtronic DBS devices and safety studies for other DBS device vendors are scarce.

Internal Pulse Generator Malfunctioning

Lastly, the magnetic fields produced by MRI could interfere with IPG function, particularly in older IPG models. Early studies using DBS devices examined patients during the "first stage" of surgery, in which the IPG has not yet been implanted and where externalized electrodes are connected to an external stimulator that remains a safe distance from the scanner via a sufficiently long cable [39, 40]. Thus, these "lead-only systems" safety studies do not provide insight on IPG function during the MRI scan. In addition, these early-stage IPG models also relied on the presence of a non-implantable transmitter near the pulse generator. Depending on the patient's position within the bore, these reed switches could spontaneously activate during scanning, which precluded the use of body-transmit coils [30]. Modern IPGs can render scanning safer by buffering eventually arising currents and transmitting them to surrounding tissues (see MRI Safety Innovations). While the newer IPG models may not have magnetic reed switches, device malfunction induced by static magnetic fields, gradients, or RF fields should nonetheless be tested following imaging as per the standards [41]. Thus far, studies featuring newer IPG models have not found IPG malfunctioning to be a risk [26].

Magnetic Resonance Imaging Safety Studies with Humans

Outside of the experimental findings conducted on phantom models, human studies have also provided insights on the safety of patients with DBS entering MR environments. The recent upsurge in human studies coincides with the end of the safety warning issued by the FDA (from 2005 to 2011) [42]. In accordance with new DBS vendor guidelines, several human studies with large cohorts were performed [37, 43–46]. None of these studies performed with a 1.5 T MRI (or at lower field strengths) reported any adverse events after scanning patients with DBS which highlighted the importance of following "on-label" guidelines recommended by vendors [43, 44].

Conversely, "off-label" studies were performed testing sequences with higher SAR, atypical IPG configurations (e.g., placed in the abdomen) [37], or higher field strengths (i.e., ≥ 3 T MRI) [34]. Indeed, as the use of 3 T MR units became more widespread, higher field strength studies did not demonstrate any adverse events across 150 patients [21, 26, 47–49]. Although these studies diverged from vendor guidelines, it must be known that it is difficult to differentiate inherent risks from lack of safety testing by implant vendors. Thus, prior to performing off-label MRI on patients with DBS, local institutional safety testing using the specific MRI hardware, DBS configuration, and sequences must be performed in phantom models. Furthermore, the integrity of the DBS device—as reflected by the device's impedances, electrical circuits, and stability of peri-electrode tissues—must be scrutinized following MRI examinations [26, 29, 48].

Special Considerations

The Impetus for Using High-Field MRI

A tremendous amount of research has been conducted using low-field (i.e., ≤ 1.5 T) MR scanners due to their clinical prevalence. Nevertheless, MR units with higher field strengths (i.e., 3 or 7 T) provide superior signal-to-noise ratio (SNR) making delineations between small abutting neural structures more apparent compared to 1.5 T [50, 51]. This improved imaging quality has the potential to provide superior diagnostics compared to lower field MR imaging. In addition, the superior SNR can reduce the number of imaging averages required to produce images, subsequently reducing the overall scan duration. However, MR scanners with higher field strengths are associated with more pronounced DBS susceptibility artifacts and geometric distortions [48]. There is a trade-off between SNR and artifact size using high-field MRI, unless techniques that reduce susceptibility artifacts are employed [48].

Depending on the field strength of the scanner and dielectric properties of a particular tissue, conductive DBS components with lengths close to the half-wavelength of the RF field have the potential for very rapid and high heating (i.e., antenna effect). 7 T MRI transmits RF pulses at a higher resonant frequency (297 MHz) than most clinical MRI field strengths (≤ 3 T), and leads to higher and more rapid temperature elevations in shorter electrically conductive implants (i.e., 5–7 cm) [25]. Furthermore, complex patterns of constructive and destructive interference created within the tissue make it difficult to produce a uniform RF transmit field within tissues at 7 T. This could foreseeably result in SAR hotspots outside of the vendor guidelines [52]. Without physical experiments and modelling of different exposure conditions (i.e., realistic MR imaging scanning, nature and location of the implants, tissue types) in the 7 T environment, direct translation of existing DBS systems could lead to significantly higher translational, or rotational forces. Recently, preliminary *ex vivo* safety testing of DBS leads disconnected and connected to the IPG within a 7 T MRI was conducted by Bhusal and colleagues found that most safety concerns (i.e., RF heating, device movement and integrity) did not pose any major risks, although more thorough, systematic assessments are required to assure all aspects of MR safety are evaluated before patients are scanned [53]. With the recent FDA approval of 7 T scanners for clinical imaging and increased accessibility at some institutions, comprehensive and rigorous safety testing (i.e., physical experiments and modelling) and risk assessments must be a customary practice, regardless of the scanner or field strength in question [54].

High-Performance Sequences

Modern MR scanners are not only increasing in field strength, but more powerful gradients are also being installed to facilitate performance enhancements (e.g., imaging with high-resolution volume, shorter echo times and echo spacing) [55, 56]. Functional magnetic resonance imaging (fMRI) sequences require such gradient performance and allow researchers to visualize brain activity changes as a result of stimulation, revealing clinically efficacious networks in DBS indications [34, 48]. A number of studies—most commonly with limitations (e.g., scanners with lower field strengths, smaller sample sizes, externalized DBS components)—have previously used fMRI to study DBS mechanisms of action. Possible safety concerns that may deter the acquisition of fMRI in DBS patients include its requirement for high-performance acquisitions (e.g., echo-planar imaging (EPI)) which may increase the risk of inducing currents, unfamiliarity with the distribution of maximum dB/dt for particular MR scanners, and the overall lack of comprehensive testing and modelling with fully-implanted systems [57]. Many researchers or clinicians likely find the additional risks unnecessary and have concerns about the data quality (i.e., susceptibility artifacts), but these concerns may be unfounded since fMRI sequences have and can be performed safely within vendor guidelines and certain imaging techniques can be applied to minimize artifacts created at higher field strengths [21, 26]. Irrespectively, many centers refrain from performing high-performance sequences due to the posed safety concerns.

Future Directions

Magnetic Resonance Safety Innovations

Technological advancements create opportunities to use techniques and tools to improve MRI safety for patients with DBS. Using phantom models poses limitations such as imprecise heating estimations. Phantom models can show considerable variation across studies due to the shape of the model and concentration of polyacrylic acid used to form the semisolid, flesh-simulating gel, along with the variations in the MR unit (i.e., hardware and software) and DBS systems (i.e., orientation and positioning) tested. In response, bioengineering innovations have emerged to improve MRI safety for patients with DBS. These innovative techniques and tools include optimized MRI acquisition parameters [58–60], modified DBS [61–63], or MRI hardware (including coils) [64–70], and computational simulation (see Fig. 5.2) [15, 71–75]. For example, DBS electrodes have even been engineered to act as heat sinks which disperse heat [64], or decrease the MRI-related susceptibility artifact [76, 77], and models using machine learning have been used to predict local SAR in tissues adjacent to the lead tips [78]. MRI hardware and coil modifications that lower SAR deposited, low-SAR MR sequence parameters that produce less electrode-related image distortions [58–60], or designing a rotatable linearly polarized birdcage transmit coil are some of the approaches different groups have taken to improve MR safety for DBS patients [79–82].

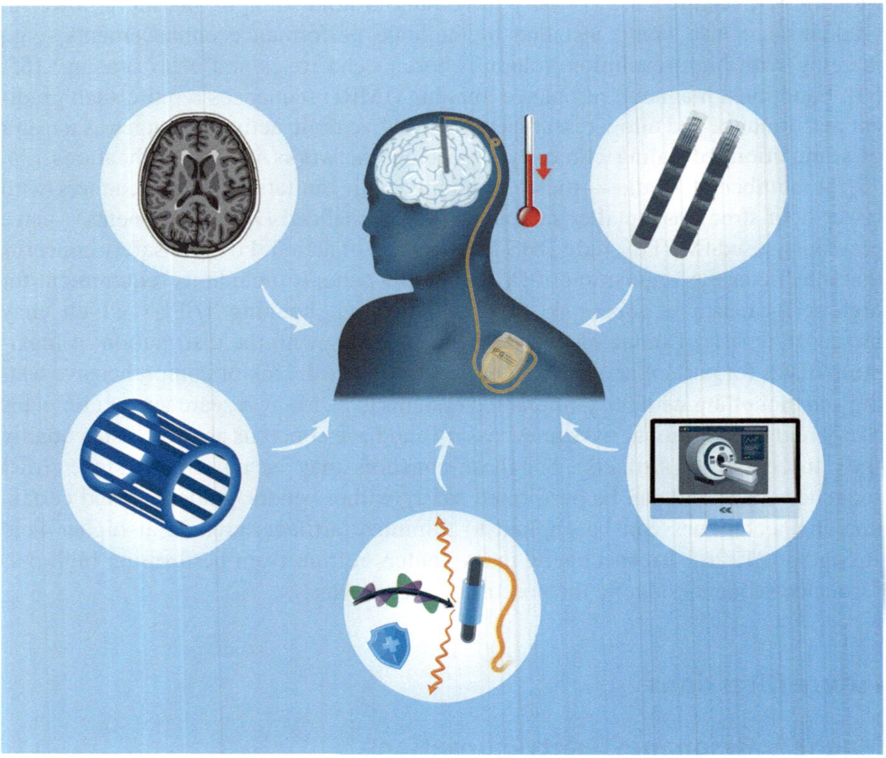

Fig. 5.2 Innovative solutions utilized to improve the safety of MRI in patients with deep brain stimulation devices. (From left to right) (i) low-specific absorption rate sequences, (ii) modifications to the magnetic resonance imaging hardware, software, and techniques (iii) use of materials or technologies to dissipate heat, (iv) computational and graphic simulators of heating, and (v) modifications to deep brain stimulation device components and lead trajectories

Substantial developments for teaching purposes have been made with a three-dimensional graphic simulator allowing for the individualization of MRI safety. In fact, one application software has been designed as an MR safety teaching tool assisting with the visualization of distributions and relative spatial strengths of the energies and magnetic fields found in different MRI scanner models [83]. Special or novel MRI cases can be simulated by the application and the patient's gender, height, weight, and implant position/orientation are accounted for [83]. Even though many of these solutions seem promising, the very complex interactions that can occur between DBS devices and MRI (in all its testing variations) still prevent us from using a robust, safe, and general solution for MRI in DBS patients.

Possibilities for a New MR Safety Process

As there are virtually no "MR Safe" AIMDs as most have metallic components, MRI scanning in DBS patients is limited by stringent guidelines. Centers should be familiar with the restrictive guidelines and use them to perform on-label scans when necessary and perform site-specific safety testing to facilitate off-label scans. Existing MR safety labels have led to early deliberations of a more open-ended process that would introduce a fourth MR classification: *MR Unlabelled* [84]. In scenarios where an MR examination is needed but the patient has a DBS device whose compatibility is unknown and the scenarios do not meet the working conditions specified for safety, the benefits must outweigh the potential risks for scanning to commence [84]. For example, if the DBS vendor MRI guidelines does not specify that the DBS Activa PC system (i.e., MR Conditional for head scans with a head-transmit/receive coil at 1.5 T) is not eligible for head-only scans at 3 T, then the device would fall under *MR Unlabelled*. Subsequently, adequate local safety risk assessment should be undertaken by a multidisciplinary team, including the MR Safety Officer, MR Safety Expert, radiologists, relevant specialists, and referring clinicians, to decide whether the study should be cancelled, or proceed under specific conditions of operation [83, 84]. The implementation of new safety processes could enable more patients with DBS indicated for an MRI to get scanned, but studies must proceed in the safest possible manner by prioritizing the health and safety of the patient and weighing the risks and benefits.

Conclusion

In summary, the complexity of factors that contribute to heating risks and other concerns have severely constrained the use of MRI in DBS patients to date. Although some institutions are exploring DBS and MRI applications following adequate safety testing that do not adhere to vendor guidelines, many other centers remain conservative and prohibit most MRI for patients with DBS. Rather than not performing MRI for patients with DBS, institutions should be familiar with the guidelines and offer, if possible, on-label scanning for clinical questions. With off-label scanning, the numerous interactions and conditions that may influence heating and other risks, observations and conclusions made at one institution are not generalizable and thus not directly applicable to other conditions or institutions regarding safety risks assessment. As with most aspects of medicine, clinicians and researchers should always weigh the risks and benefits of conducting off-label interventions and this decision should not solely be dictated by a label or mark. Only if MRI is likely to provide substantial benefits for the patient with DBS and considerable local safety testing and risk assessments have been performed, then some degree of risk may be justified.

Acknowledgement We would like to express our gratitude to Yu-Ming Chang, our illustrator, for his work on all the figures depicted in this chapter.

References

1. Falowski S, Safriel Y, Ryan MP, Hargens L. The rate of magnetic resonance imaging in patients with deep brain stimulation. Stereotact Funct Neurosurg. 2016;94(3):147–53. https://doi.org/10.1159/000444760. Epub 20160601. Cited in: Pubmed; PMID 27245875
2. Paff M, Loh A, Sarica C, Lozano AM, Fasano A. Update on current technologies for deep brain stimulation in Parkinson's disease. J Mov Disord. 2020;13(3):185–98. https://doi.org/10.14802/jmd.20052. Epub 20200831. Cited in: Pubmed; PMID 32854482
3. Shellock FG. Magnetic resonance safety update 2002: implants and devices. J Magn Reson Imaging. 2002;16(5):485–96. https://doi.org/10.1002/jmri.10196. Cited in: Pubmed; PMID 12412025
4. Coffey RJ. Deep brain stimulation devices: a brief technical history and review. Artif Organs. 2009;33(3):208–20. https://doi.org/10.1111/j.1525-1594.2008.00620.x. Epub 20080731 Cited in: Pubmed; PMID 18684199
5. Elster AD, Link KM, Carr JJ. Patient screening prior to MR imaging: a practical approach synthesized from protocols at 15 U. S. medical centers. Am J Roentgenol. 1994;162(1):195–9. https://doi.org/10.2214/ajr.162.1.8273665.
6. Spiegel J, Fuss G, Backens M, Reith W, Magnus T, Becker G, Moringlane JR, Dillmann U. Transient dystonia following magnetic resonance imaging in a patient with deep brain stimulation electrodes for the treatment of Parkinson disease. Case report. J Neurosurg. 2003;99(4):772–4. https://doi.org/10.3171/jns.2003.99.4.0772. Cited in: Pubmed; PMID 14567615
7. Henderson JM, Tkach J, Phillips M, Baker K, Shellock FG, Rezai AR. Permanent neurological deficit related to magnetic resonance imaging in a patient with implanted deep brain stimulation electrodes for Parkinson's disease: case report. Neurosurgery. 2005;57(5):E1063. https://doi.org/10.1227/01.neu.0000180810.16964.3e. discussion E1063. Cited in: Pubmed; PMID 16284543
8. Zrinzo L, Yoshida F, Hariz MI, Thornton J, Foltynie T, Yousry TA, Limousin P. Clinical safety of brain magnetic resonance imaging with implanted deep brain stimulation hardware: large case series and review of the literature. World Neurosurg. 2011;76(1-2):164–72. https://doi.org/10.1016/j.wneu.2011.02.029. discussion 69–73. Cited in: Pubmed; PMID 21839969
9. (ASTM) ASfTaM. ASTM F2182-19e2, Standard Test Method for Measurement of Radio Frequency Induced Heating On or Near Passive Implants During Magnetic Resonance Imaging. West Conshohocken, Pa; 2020. ASTM International.
10. Stafford RJ. The physics of magnetic resonance imaging safety. Magn Reson Imaging Clin N Am. 2020;28(4):517–36. https://doi.org/10.1016/j.mric.2020.08.002. 2020/11/01/

11. Erhardt JB, Fuhrer E, Gruschke OG, Leupold J, Wapler MC, Hennig J, Stieglitz T, Korvink JG. Should patients with brain implants undergo MRI? J Neural Eng. 2018;15(4):041002. https://doi.org/10.1088/1741-2552/aab4e4. Epub 20180307. Cited in: Pubmed; PMID 29513262
12. Delfino JG, Woods TO. New developments in standards for MRI safety testing of medical devices. Curr Radiol Rep. 2016;4(6):28. https://doi.org/10.1007/s40134-016-0155-y.
13. (ISO/TS) IOfSTS. 10974, Assessment of the safety of magnetic resonance imaging for patients with an active implantable medical device. 2 ed. Geneva, Switzerland; 2018. Report No. ISO/TS 10974. International Organization for Standardization.
14. (IEC) IEC. 60601-2-33, Medical electrical equipment - Part 2-33: Particular requirements for the basic safety and essential performance of magnetic resonance equipment for medical diagnosis. Geneva, Switzerland; 2010. IEC.
15. Golestanirad L, Kirsch J, Bonmassar G, Downs S, Elahi B, Martin A, Iacono MI, Angelone LM, Keil B, Wald LL, Pilitsis J. RF-induced heating in tissue near bilateral DBS implants during MRI at 1.5T and 3T: the role of surgical lead management. NeuroImage. 2019;184:566–76. Epub 20180919. https://doi.org/10.1016/j.neuroimage.2018.09.034. Cited in: Pubmed; PMID 30243973
16. Baker KB, Tkach J, Hall JD, Nyenhuis JA, Shellock FG, Rezai AR. Reduction of magnetic resonance imaging-related heating in deep brain stimulation leads using a lead management device. Neurosurgery. 2005;57(4 Suppl):392–7.; Cited in: Pubmed; PMID 16234691 discussion 392–7. https://doi.org/10.1227/01.neu.0000176877.26994.0c.
17. Rezai AR, Finelli D, Nyenhuis JA, Hrdlicka G, Tkach J, Sharan A, Rugieri P, Stypulkowski PH, Shellock FG. Neurostimulation systems for deep brain stimulation: in vitro evaluation of magnetic resonance imaging-related heating at 1.5 tesla. J Magn Reson Imaging. 2002;15(3):241–50. https://doi.org/10.1002/jmri.10069. Cited in: Pubmed; PMID 11891968
18. Nazzaro JM, Klemp JA, Brooks WM, Cook-Wiens G, Mayo MS, Van Acker GM 3rd, Lyons KE, Cheney PD. Deep brain stimulation lead-contact heating during 3T MRI: single- versus dual-channel pulse generator configurations. Int J Neurosci. 2014;124(3):166–74. Epub 20131008. Cited in: Pubmed; PMID 24000873. https://doi.org/10.3109/00207454.2013.840303.
19. Morishita T, Hilliard JD, Okun MS, Neal D, Nestor KA, Peace D, Hozouri AA, Davidson MR, Bova FJ, Sporrer JM, Oyama G, Foote KD. Postoperative lead migration in deep brain stimulation surgery: incidence, risk factors, and clinical impact. PLoS One. 2017;12(9):e0183711. https://doi.org/10.1371/journal.pone.0183711. Epub 20170913. Cited in: Pubmed; PMID 28902876
20. Dempsey MF, Condon B. Thermal injuries associated with MRI. Clin Radiol. 2001;56(6):457–65. https://doi.org/10.1053/crad.2000.0688. Cited in: Pubmed; PMID 11428795
21. Hancu I, Boutet A, Fiveland E, Ranjan M, Prusik J, Dimarzio M, Rashid T, Ashe J, Xu D, Kalia SK, Hodaie M, Fasano A, Kucharczyk W, Pilitsis J, Lozano A, Madhavan R. On the (non-)equivalency of monopolar and bipolar settings for deep brain stimulation fMRI studies of Parkinson's disease patients. J Magn Reson Imaging. 2019;49(6):1736–49. https://doi.org/10.1002/jmri.26321. Epub 20181215. Cited in: Pubmed; PMID 30552842
22. Kahan J, Papadaki A, White M, Mancini L, Yousry T, Zrinzo L, Limousin P, Hariz M, Foltynie T, Thornton J. The safety of using body-transmit MRI in patients with implanted deep brain stimulation devices. PLoS One. 2015;10(6):e0129077. https://doi.org/10.1371/journal.pone.0129077. Epub 20150610. Cited in: Pubmed; PMID 26061738
23. Baker KB, Tkach JA, Nyenhuis JA, Phillips M, Shellock FG, Gonzalez-Martinez J, Rezai AR. Evaluation of specific absorption rate as a dosimeter of MRI-related implant heating. J Magn Reson Imaging. 2004;20(2):315–20. https://doi.org/10.1002/jmri.20103. Cited in: Pubmed; PMID 15269959
24. Baker KB, Tkach JA, Phillips MD, Rezai AR. Variability in RF-induced heating of a deep brain stimulation implant across MR systems. J Magn Reson Imaging. 2006;24(6):1236–42. https://doi.org/10.1002/jmri.20769. Cited in: Pubmed; PMID 17078088
25. Zheng J, Xia M, Kainz W, Chen J. Wire-based sternal closure: MRI-related heating at 1.5 T/64 MHz and 3 T/128 MHz based on simulation and experimental phantom study. Magn

Reson Med. 2020;83(3):1055–65. https://doi.org/10.1002/mrm.27963. Epub 20190829. Cited in: Pubmed; PMID 31468593

26. Boutet A, Hancu I, Saha U, Crawley A, Xu DS, Ranjan M, Hlasny E, Chen R, Foltz W, Sammartino F, Coblentz A, Kucharczyk W, Lozano AM. 3-tesla MRI of deep brain stimulation patients: safety assessment of coils and pulse sequences. J Neurosurg. 2019;132(2):586–94. https://doi.org/10.3171/2018.11.JNS181338. Cited in: Pubmed; PMID 30797197
27. Mayberg HS, Lozano AM, Voon V, McNeely HE, Seminowicz D, Hamani C, Schwalb JM, Kennedy SH. Deep brain stimulation for treatment-resistant depression. Neuron. 2005;45(5):651–60. https://doi.org/10.1016/j.neuron.2005.02.014. Cited in: Pubmed; PMID 15748841
28. Carmichael DW, Pinto S, Limousin-Dowsey P, Thobois S, Allen PJ, Lemieux L, Yousry T, Thornton JS. Functional MRI with active, fully implanted, deep brain stimulation systems: safety and experimental confounds. NeuroImage. 2007;37(2):508–17. https://doi.org/10.1016/j.neuroimage.2007.04.058. Cited in: Pubmed; PMID 17590355 Epub 20070518
29. Georgi JC, Stippich C, Tronnier VM, Heiland S. Active deep brain stimulation during MRI: a feasibility study. Magn Reson Med. 2004;51(2):380–8. https://doi.org/10.1002/mrm.10699. Cited in: Pubmed; PMID 14755664
30. Gleason CA, Kaula NF, Hricak H, Schmidt RA, Tanagho EA. The effect of magnetic resonance imagers on implanted neurostimulators. Pacing Clin Electrophysiol. 1992;15(1):81–94. https://doi.org/10.1111/j.1540-8159.1992.tb02904.x. Cited in: Pubmed; PMID 1371004
31. Bhavaraju NC, Nagaraddi V, Chetlapalli SR, Osorio I. Electrical and thermal behavior of non-ferrous noble metal electrodes exposed to MRI fields. Magn Reson Imaging. 2002;20(4):351–7. https://doi.org/10.1016/S0730-725X(02)00506-4.
32. Bhidayasiri R, Bronstein JM, Sinha S, Krahl SE, Ahn S, Behnke EJ, Cohen MS, Frysinger R, Shellock FG. Bilateral neurostimulation systems used for deep brain stimulation: in vitro study of MRI-related heating at 1.5 T and implications for clinical imaging of the brain. Magn Reson Imaging. 2005;23(4):549–55. https://doi.org/10.1016/j.mri.2005.02.007. Cited in: Pubmed; PMID 15919600
33. Finelli DA, Rezai AR, Ruggieri PM, Tkach JA, Nyenhuis JA, Hrdlicka G, Sharan A, Gonzalez-Martinez J, Stypulkowski PH, Shellock FG. MR imaging-related heating of deep brain stimulation electrodes: in vitro study. AJNR Am J Neuroradiol. 2002;23(10):1795–802. Cited in: Pubmed; PMID 12427641
34. Phillips MD, Baker KB, Lowe MJ, Tkach JA, Cooper SE, Kopell BH, Rezai AR. Parkinson disease: pattern of functional MR imaging activation during deep brain stimulation of subthalamic nucleus—initial experience. Radiology. 2006;239(1):209–16. https://doi.org/10.1148/radiol.2391041990. Cited in: Pubmed; PMID 16567487
35. Park SM, Nyenhuis JA, Smith CD, Lim EJ, Foster KS, Baker KB, Hrdlicka G, Rezai AR, Ruggieri P, Sharan A, Shellock FG, Stypulkowski PH, Tkach J. Gelled versus nongelled phantom material for measurement of MRI-induced temperature increases with bioimplants. IEEE Trans Magn. 2003;39(5):3367–71. https://doi.org/10.1109/TMAG.2003.816259.
36. Kainz W, Neubauer G, Uberbacher R, Alesch F, Chan DD. Temperature measurement on neurological pulse generators during MR scans. Biomed Eng Online. 2002;1:2. https://doi.org/10.1186/1475-925x-1-2. Cited in: Pubmed; PMID 12437766 . Epub 20020912
37. Nazzaro JM, Lyons KE, Wetzel LH, Pahwa R. Use of brain MRI after deep brain stimulation hardware implantation. Int J Neurosci. 2010;120(3):176–83. https://doi.org/10.3109/00207450903389156. Cited in: Pubmed; PMID 20374084
38. Schueler BA, Parrish TB, Lin JC, Hammer BE, Pangrle BJ, Ritenour ER, Kucharczyk J, Truwit CL. MRI compatibility and visibility assessment of implantable medical devices. J Magn Reson Imaging. 1999;9(4):596–603. https://doi.org/10.1002/(sici)1522-2586(199904)9:4<596::aid-jmri14>3.0.co;2-t. Cited in: Pubmed; PMID 10232520
39. Sarem-Aslani A, Mullett K. Industrial perspective on deep brain stimulation: history, current state, and future developments. Front Integr Neurosci. 2011;5:46. Epub 20110927. https://doi.org/10.3389/fnint.2011.00046. Cited in: Pubmed; PMID 21991248

40. Jech R, Mueller K. Investigating network effects of DBS with fMRI. In: Horn A, editor. Connectomic deep brain stimulation. Academic Press; 2022. p. 275–301.
41. (ASTM) ASfTaM. ASTM F2052-15, Standard Test Method for Measurement of Magnetically Induced Displacement Force on Medical Devices in the Magnetic Resonance Environment. West Conshohocken, Pa; 2018. ASTM International.
42. Boutet A, Chow CT, Narang K, Elias GJB, Neudorfer C, Germann J, Ranjan M, Loh A, Martin AJ, Kucharczyk W, Steele CJ, Hancu I, Rezai AR, Lozano AM. Improving safety of MRI in patients with deep brain stimulation devices. Radiology. 2020;296(2):250–62. https://doi.org/10.1148/radiol.2020192291. Epub 20200623 Cited in: Pubmed; PMID 32573388
43. Larson PS, Richardson RM, Starr PA, Martin AJ. Magnetic resonance imaging of implanted deep brain stimulators: experience in a large series. Stereotact Funct Neurosurg. 2008;86(2):92–100. https://doi.org/10.1159/000112430. Epub 20071212. Cited in: Pubmed; PMID 18073522
44. Tagliati M, Jankovic J, Pagan F, Susatia F, Isaias IU, Okun MS, National Parkinson Foundation DBSWG. Safety of MRI in patients with implanted deep brain stimulation devices. NeuroImage. 2009;47(Suppl 2):T53–7. https://doi.org/10.1016/j.neuroimage.2009.04.044. Epub 20090417. Cited in: Pubmed; PMID 19376247
45. Chhabra V, Sung E, Mewes K, Bakay RA, Abosch A, Gross RE. Safety of magnetic resonance imaging of deep brain stimulator systems: a serial imaging and clinical retrospective study. J Neurosurg. 2010;112(3):497–502. https://doi.org/10.3171/2009.7.JNS09572. Cited in: Pubmed; PMID 19681685
46. Fraix V, Chabardes S, Krainik A, Seigneuret E, Grand S, Le Bas JF, Krack P, Benabid AL, Pollak P. Effects of magnetic resonance imaging in patients with implanted deep brain stimulation systems. J Neurosurg. 2010;113(6):1242–5. https://doi.org/10.3171/2010.1.JNS09951. Epub 20100226. Cited in: Pubmed; PMID 20187699
47. Sammartino F, Krishna V, Sankar T, Fisico J, Kalia SK, Hodaie M, Kucharczyk W, Mikulis DJ, Crawley A, Lozano AM. 3-tesla MRI in patients with fully implanted deep brain stimulation devices: a preliminary study in 10 patients. J Neurosurg. 2017;127(4):892–8. https://doi.org/10.3171/2016.9.JNS16908. Epub 20161223. Cited in: Pubmed; PMID 28009238
48. Boutet A, Rashid T, Hancu I, Elias GJB, Gramer RM, Germann J, Dimarzio M, Li B, Paramanandam V, Prasad S, Ranjan M, Coblentz A, Gwun D, Chow CT, Maciel R, Soh D, Fiveland E, Hodaie M, Kalia SK, Fasano A, Kucharczyk W, Pilitsis J, Lozano AM. Functional MRI safety and artifacts during deep brain stimulation: experience in 102 patients. Radiology. 2019;293(1):174–83. https://doi.org/10.1148/radiol.2019190546. Epub 20190806. Cited in: Pubmed; PMID 31385756
49. DiMarzio M, Rashid T, Hancu I, Fiveland E, Prusik J, Gillogly M, Madhavan R, Joel S, Durphy J, Molho E, Hanspal E, Shin D, Pilitsis JG. Functional MRI signature of chronic pain relief from deep brain stimulation in Parkinson disease patients. Neurosurgery. 2019;85(6):E1043–9. https://doi.org/10.1093/neuros/nyz269. Cited in: Pubmed; PMID 31313816
50. Maubon AJ, Ferru JM, Berger V, Soulage MC, DeGraef M, Aubas P, Coupeau P, Dumont E, Rouanet JP. Effect of field strength on MR images: comparison of the same subject at 0.5, 1.0, and 1.5 T. Radiographics. 1999;19(4):1057–67. https://doi.org/10.1148/radiographics.19.4.g99jl281057. Cited in: Pubmed; PMID 10464808
51. Collins CM, Smith MB. Signal-to-noise ratio and absorbed power as functions of main magnetic field strength, and definition of "90 degrees " RF pulse for the head in the birdcage coil. Magn Reson Med. 2001;45(4):684–91. https://doi.org/10.1002/mrm.1091. Cited in: Pubmed; PMID 11283997
52. Fagan AJ, Amrami KK, Welker KM, Frick MA, Felmlee JP, Watson RE. Magnetic resonance safety in the 7T environment. Magn Reson Imaging Clin N Am. 2020;28(4):573–82. https://doi.org/10.1016/j.mric.2020.07.002.
53. Bhusal B, Stockmann J, Guerin B, Mareyam A, Kirsch J, Wald LL, Nolt MJ, Rosenow J, Lopez-Rosado R, Elahi B, Golestanirad L. Safety and image quality at 7T MRI for deep brain stimulation systems: ex vivo study with lead-only and full-systems. PLoS One. 2021;16(9):e0257077.

https://doi.org/10.1371/journal.pone.0257077. The authors have declared that no competing interests exist. Epub 20210907 Cited in: Pubmed; PMID 34492090

54. Burkett BJ, Fagan AJ, Felmlee JP, Black DF, Lane JI, Port JD, Rydberg CH, Welker KM. Clinical 7-T MRI for neuroradiology: strengths, weaknesses, and ongoing challenges. Neuroradiology. 2021;63(2):167–77. https://doi.org/10.1007/s00234-020-02629-z Epub 20210102. Cited in: Pubmed; PMID 33388947
55. Okada T, Yamada H, Ito H, Yonekura Y, Sadato N. Magnetic field strength increase yields significantly greater contrast-to-noise ratio increase: measured using BOLD contrast in the primary visual area. Acad Radiol. 2005;12(2):142–7. https://doi.org/10.1016/j.acra.2004.11.012. Cited in: Pubmed; PMID 15721590
56. Olman CA, Yacoub E. High-field FMRI for human applications: an overview of spatial resolution and signal specificity. Open Neuroimaging J. 2011;5:74–89. https://doi.org/10.2174/1874440001105010074. Epub 20111104. Cited in: Pubmed; PMID 22216080
57. Poustchi-Amin M, Mirowitz SA, Brown JJ, McKinstry RC, Li T. Principles and applications of echo-planar imaging: a review for the general radiologist. Radiographics. 2001;21(3):767–79. https://doi.org/10.1148/radiographics.21.3.g01ma23767. Cited in: Pubmed; PMID 11353123
58. Sarkar SN, Papavassiliou E, Hackney DB, Alsop DC, Shih LC, Madhuranthakam AJ, Busse RF, La Ruche S, Bhadelia RA. Three-dimensional brain MRI for DBS patients within ultra-low radiofrequency power limits. Mov Disord. 2014;29(4):546–9. https://doi.org/10.1002/mds.25808. Epub 20140117. Cited in: Pubmed; PMID 24442797
59. Sarkar SN, Papavassiliou E, Rojas R, Teich DL, Hackney DB, Bhadelia RA, Stormann J, Alterman RL. Low-power inversion recovery MRI preserves brain tissue contrast for patients with Parkinson disease with deep brain stimulators. AJNR Am J Neuroradiol. 2014;35(7):1325–9. https://doi.org/10.3174/ajnr.A3896. Epub 20140327. Cited in: Pubmed; PMID 24676004
60. Sarkar SN, Sarkar PR, Papavassiliou E, Rojas RR. Utilizing fast spin echo MRI to reduce image artifacts and improve implant/tissue interface detection in refractory Parkinson's patients with deep brain stimulators. Parkinsons Dis. 2014;2014:508576. https://doi.org/10.1155/2014/508576. Epub 20140225. Cited in: Pubmed; PMID 24724036
61. Elwassif MM, Datta A, Rahman A, Bikson M. Temperature control at DBS electrodes using a heat sink: experimentally validated FEM model of DBS lead architecture. J Neural Eng. 2012;9(4):046009. https://doi.org/10.1088/1741-2560/9/4/046009. Epub 20120704. Cited in: Pubmed; PMID 22764359
62. Serano P, Angelone LM, Katnani H, Eskandar E, Bonmassar G. A novel brain stimulation technology provides compatibility with MRI. Sci Rep. 2015;5:9805. https://doi.org/10.1038/srep09805. Epub 20150429. Cited in: Pubmed; PMID 25924189
63. Golestanirad L, Angelone LM, Kirsch J, Downs S, Keil B, Bonmassar G, Wald LL. Reducing RF-induced heating near implanted leads through high-dielectric capacitive bleeding of current (CBLOC). IEEE Trans Microw Theory Tech. 2019;67(3):1265–73. https://doi.org/10.1109/TMTT.2018.2885517. Epub 20190101. Cited in: Pubmed; PMID 31607756
64. Eryaman Y, Guerin B, Akgun C, Herraiz JL, Martin A, Torrado-Carvajal A, Malpica N, Hernandez-Tamames JA, Schiavi E, Adalsteinsson E, Wald LL. Parallel transmit pulse design for patients with deep brain stimulation implants. Magn Reson Med. 2015;73(5):1896–903. https://doi.org/10.1002/mrm.25324. Epub 20140619 Cited in: Pubmed; PMID 24947104
65. Gudino N, Sonmez M, Yao Z, Baig T, Nielles-Vallespin S, Faranesh AZ, Lederman RJ, Martens M, Balaban RS, Hansen MS, Griswold MA. Parallel transmit excitation at 1.5 T based on the minimization of a driving function for device heating. Med Phys. 2015;42(1):359–71. https://doi.org/10.1118/1.4903894. Cited in: Pubmed; PMID 25563276
66. McElcheran CE, Golestanirad L, Iacono MI, Wei PS, Yang B, Anderson KJT, Bonmassar G, Graham SJ. Numerical simulations of realistic Lead trajectories and an experimental verification support the efficacy of parallel radiofrequency transmission to reduce heating of deep brain stimulation implants during MRI. Sci Rep. 2019;9(1):2124. https://doi.org/10.1038/s41598-018-38099-w. Cited in: Pubmed; PMID 30765724. Epub 20190214.

67. McElcheran CE, Yang B, Anderson KJT, Golestanirad L, Graham SJ. Parallel radiofrequency transmission at 3 tesla to improve safety in bilateral implanted wires in a heterogeneous model. Magn Reson Med. 2017;78(6):2406–15. https://doi.org/10.1002/mrm.26622. Epub 20170228. Cited in: Pubmed; PMID 28244142
68. McElcheran CE, Yang B, Anderson KJ, Golenstani-Rad L, Graham SJ. Investigation of parallel radiofrequency transmission for the reduction of heating in long conductive leads in 3 tesla magnetic resonance imaging. PLoS One. 2015;10(8):e0134379. https://doi.org/10.1371/journal.pone.0134379. Epub 20150803. Cited in: Pubmed; PMID 26237218
69. Eryaman Y, Kobayashi N, Moen S, Aman J, Grant A, Vaughan JT, Molnar G, Park MC, Vitek J, Adriany G, Ugurbil K, Harel N. A simple geometric analysis method for measuring and mitigating RF induced currents on deep brain stimulation leads by multichannel transmission/reception. NeuroImage. 2019;184:658–68. https://doi.org/10.1016/j.neuroimage.2018.09.072. Epub 20180928. Cited in: Pubmed; PMID 30273715
70. Guerin B, Angelone LM, Dougherty D, Wald LL. Parallel transmission to reduce absorbed power around deep brain stimulation devices in MRI: impact of number and arrangement of transmit channels. Magn Reson Med. 2020;83(1):299–311. https://doi.org/10.1002/mrm.27905. Epub 20190807 Cited in: Pubmed; PMID 31389069
71. Golombeck MA, Thiele J, Dossel O. Magnetic resonance imaging with implanted neurostimulators: numerical calculation of the induced heating. Biomed Tech (Berl). 2002;47(Suppl 1 Pt 2):660–3. https://doi.org/10.1515/bmte.2002.47.s1b.660. Cited in: Pubmed; PMID 12465267
72. Angelone LM, Ahveninen J, Belliveau JW, Bonmassar G. Analysis of the role of lead resistivity in specific absorption rate for deep brain stimulator leads at 3T MRI. IEEE Trans Med Imaging. 2010;29(4):1029–38. https://doi.org/10.1109/TMI.2010.2040624. Epub 20100322 Cited in: Pubmed; PMID 20335090
73. Iacono MI, Makris N, Mainardi L, Angelone LM, Bonmassar G. MRI-based multiscale model for electromagnetic analysis in the human head with implanted DBS. Comput Math Methods Med. 2013;2013:694171. https://doi.org/10.1155/2013/694171. Epub 20130715. Cited in: Pubmed; PMID 23956789
74. Bonmassar G, Angelone LM, Makris N. A virtual patient simulator based on human connectome and 7 T MRI for deep brain stimulation. Int J Adv Life Sci. 2014 6(3-4):364–72. Cited in: Pubmed; PMID 25705324
75. Guerin B, Serano P, Iacono MI, Herrington TM, Widge AS, Dougherty DD, Bonmassar G, Angelone LM, Wald LL. Realistic modeling of deep brain stimulation implants for electromagnetic MRI safety studies. Phys Med Biol. 2018;63(9):095015. https://doi.org/10.1088/1361-6560/aabd50. Epub 20180504. Cited in: Pubmed; PMID 29637905
76. Lai HY, Albaugh DL, Kao YC, Younce JR, Shih YY. Robust deep brain stimulation functional MRI procedures in rats and mice using an MR-compatible tungsten microwire electrode. Magn Reson Med. 2015;73(3):1246–51. https://doi.org/10.1002/mrm.25239. Epub 20140505 Cited in: Pubmed; PMID 24798216
77. Zhao S, Liu X, Xu Z, Ren H, Deng B, Tang M, Lu L, Fu X, Peng H, Liu Z, Duan X. Graphene encapsulated copper microwires as highly MRI compatible Neural electrodes. Nano Lett. 2016;16(12):7731–8. https://doi.org/10.1021/acs.nanolett.6b03829. Epub 20161117. Cited in: Pubmed; PMID 27802387
78. Vu J, Nguyen BT, Bhusal B, Baraboo J, Rosenow J, Bagci U, Bright MG, Golestanirad L. Machine learning-based prediction of MRI-induced power absorption in the tissue in patients with simplified deep brain stimulation lead models. IEEE Trans Electromagn Compat. 2021;63(5):1757–66. https://doi.org/10.1109/TEMC.2021.3106872.
79. Golestanirad L, Iacono MI, Keil B, Angelone LM, Bonmassar G, Fox MD, Herrington T, Adalsteinsson E, LaPierre C, Mareyam A, Wald LL. Construction and modeling of a reconfigurable MRI coil for lowering SAR in patients with deep brain stimulation implants. NeuroImage. 2017;147:577–88. https://doi.org/10.1016/j.neuroimage.2016.12.056. Epub 20161221. Cited in: Pubmed; PMID 28011252
80. Golestanirad L, Kazemivalipour E, Keil B, Downs S, Kirsch J, Elahi B, Pilitsis J, Wald LL. Reconfigurable MRI coil technology can substantially reduce RF heating of deep brain

stimulation implants: first in-vitro study of RF heating reduction in bilateral DBS leads at 1.5 T. PLoS One. 2019;14(8):e0220043. https://doi.org/10.1371/journal.pone.0220043. The authors have declared that no competing interests exist. Epub 20190807. Cited in: Pubmed; PMID 31390346

81. Golestanirad L, Keil B, Angelone LM, Bonmassar G, Mareyam A, Wald LL. Feasibility of using linearly polarized rotating birdcage transmitters and close-fitting receive arrays in MRI to reduce SAR in the vicinity of deep brain simulation implants. Magn Reson Med. 2017;77(4):1701–12. https://doi.org/10.1002/mrm.26220. Epub 20160405. Cited in: Pubmed; PMID 27059266
82. Kazemivalipour E, Keil B, Vali A, Rajan S, Elahi B, Atalar E, Wald LL, Rosenow J, Pilitsis J, Golestanirad L. Reconfigurable MRI technology for low-SAR imaging of deep brain stimulation at 3T: application in bilateral leads, fully-implanted systems, and surgically modified lead trajectories. NeuroImage. 2019;199:18–29. https://doi.org/10.1016/j.neuroimage.2019.05.015. Epub 20190513. Cited in: Pubmed; PMID 31096058
83. Kanal E. Standardized approaches to MR safety assessment of patients with implanted devices. Magn Reson Imaging Clin N Am. 2020;28(4):537–48. https://doi.org/10.1016/j.mric.2020.07.003.
84. (MHRA) MaHPRA. Safety guidelines for magnetic resonance imaging equipment in clinical use. 4 ed.; 2021. MHRA.

Postoperative MRI Applications in Patients with DBS

6

Jürgen Germann, Flavia V. Gouveia, Emily H. Y. Wong, and Andreas Horn

Introduction

There are several applications for postoperative Magnetic Resonance Imaging (MRI) in Deep Brain Stimulation (DBS) patients that are important for both clinical practice and research. DBS utilises precisely placed electrodes to deliver carefully titrated electrical stimulation to modulate dysfunctional brain circuits [1, 2]. Confirmation of electrode placement after the surgery can be done using MRI or Computed Tomography (CT). Accurate electrode placement is crucial for clinical

J. Germann (✉) · E. H. Y. Wong
Division of Neurosurgery, Department of Surgery, University Health Network and University of Toronto, Toronto, ON, Canada

Toronto Western Hospital, University Health Network, Toronto, ON, Canada
e-mail: jurgen.germann@uhnresearch.ca

F. V. Gouveia
Neuroscience and Mental Health, Hospital for Sick Children Research Institute, Toronto, ON, Canada

A. Horn
Movement Disorders & Neuromodulation Unit, Department for Neurology, Charité – University Medicine, Berlin, Germany

Center for Brain Circuit Therapeutics, Department of Neurology, Brigham & Women's Hospital, Harvard Medical School, Boston, MA, USA

Massachusetts General Hospital Neurosurgery, Center for Neurotechnology and Neurorecovery, Massachusetts General Hospital, Harvard Medical School, Boston, MA, USA
e-mail: AHORN1@bwh.harvard.edu

A. Boutet, A. M. Lozano (eds.), *Magnetic Resonance Imaging in Deep Brain Stimulation*, https://doi.org/10.1007/978-3-031-16348-7_6

benefit as misplacement by as little as 2 mm can result in poor outcome and might necessitate a second surgery to correct electrode position [3, 4]. Investigating the relationship between individual electrode location, determined using pre- and post-operative imaging, and clinical outcome across multiple patients can be used to investigate optimal location for electrode placements, so-called 'sweet spots' of DBS stimulation [5–9]. Knowing the exact electrode trajectory and location also allows to precisely map electrophysiological data providing insights into physiological characteristics, possible disease processes, and the effects of electrical stimulation to specific brain regions [10–12]. Furthermore, MRI lead placement combined with whole brain functional or structural MRI data can be used to elucidate the brain wide networks implicated in symptom improvement following DBS treatment [5, 13–16]. Lastly, post-surgical structural MRI acquired at various intervals, either for research purposes or because they were clinically indicated can also be used to assess longitudinal structural changes providing insight into long-term changes associated with the clinical effect of DBS stimulation [17].

Electrode Localisation and Mapping of Optimal DBS Target Using Pre- and Postoperative Imaging

Multiple studies have demonstrated that optimal clinical benefit of DBS treatment is related to precise electrode placement, on the order of millimetres [5–7, 16, 18–20]. These studies make use of the small variability in exact electrode placement found across large cohorts to allow the determination of the optimal treatment target in terms of anatomical location, a process referred to as 'sweet spot mapping' [9]. It is imperative for these techniques that the patients' electrodes are localised precisely and that the electrical field induced by the individual stimulation is modelled faithfully. Moreover, steps of making localisations comparable—across patients or even DBS centres and surgeons—are needed. This often involves registering electrodes to a common model of the target structure, such as a model STN [21]. Practically speaking, most researchers currently choose to register data into a commonly used stereotactic standard brain template defined by the Montreal Neurological Institute (MNI space).

Either CT or MRI can be used to visualise the DBS electrode postoperatively (Fig. 6.1). These postoperative images are then registered to (i.e., MRI) or fused with (i.e., CT) the preoperative MRI to localise the lead precisely. Fusing postoperative CT images with the corresponding preoperative MRI has proven successful for lead localisation [22] and using postoperative CT offers the advantage that the artefact is slightly smaller compared to postoperative MRI and higher signal-to-noise in the electrode artefact [23, 24]. However, using postoperative MR images offers some distinct advantages: MRI uses non-ionising radiation, allows for the detection of complications such as infarctions [25–28], and the better anatomical contrast enables fine-scale registration with the preoperative image that will allow for the detection and correction of possible local brain shifts [29, 30]. While it has been suggested that spatial distortion deteriorates the precision of the metallic artefact on MRI [31, 32], subsequent studies have demonstrated that the artefact is a reliable

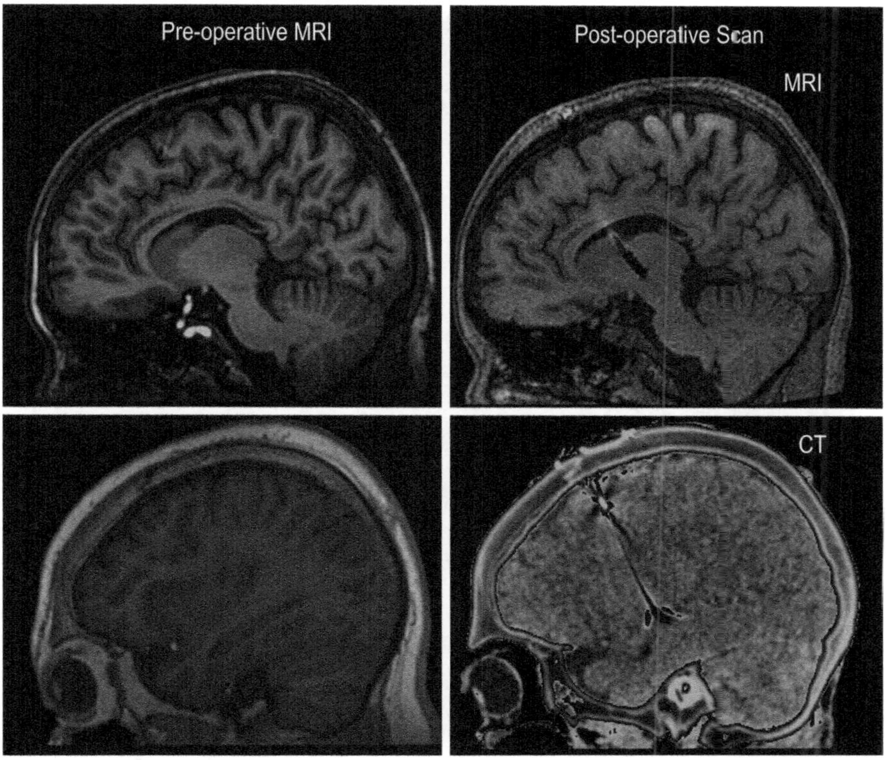

Fig. 6.1 Lead localisation using Magnetic Resonance Imaging (MRI) or Computed Tomography (CT). Top row shows a sagittal preoperative MRI on the left and the corresponding postoperative MRI on the right. The hypointense MRI artefact corresponds to the Deep Brain Stimulation (DBS) lead. The lead contacts cause a slightly enlarged artefact allowing for direct localisation. Bottom row shows a sagittal preoperative MRI on the left and the corresponding postoperative CT on the right. The DBS causes a metallic artefact (hyperintense in plane, hypointense elsewhere). *MRI* Magnetic Resonance Imaging, *CT* Computed Tomography

marker of lead localisation [33]. Furthermore, the theoretical advantage in precision of CT as compared to MRI is small and can be further minimised by optimising postoperative MRI acquisition [34, 35]. Multiple studies have demonstrated that DBS electrodes can be localised with high precision using postoperative MRI (Fig. 6.2) [3, 28, 34]. Also, MRI offers the opportunity to safely use various specialised sequences with implanted leads that allow for direct target visualisation, and thus precise estimation of anatomical lead placement [36–41]. A recent study suggests that MRI-assisted direct targeting might allow comparable individual precision in lead placement as the use of intraoperative microelectrode recordings [42] and direct MRI-based targeting is a concept highly debated and actively being investigated, especially in light of improvements in imaging resolution.

Once the DBS lead is localised successfully, sophisticated modelling can be applied to determine the Volume of Activated Tissue (VAT; also sometimes called

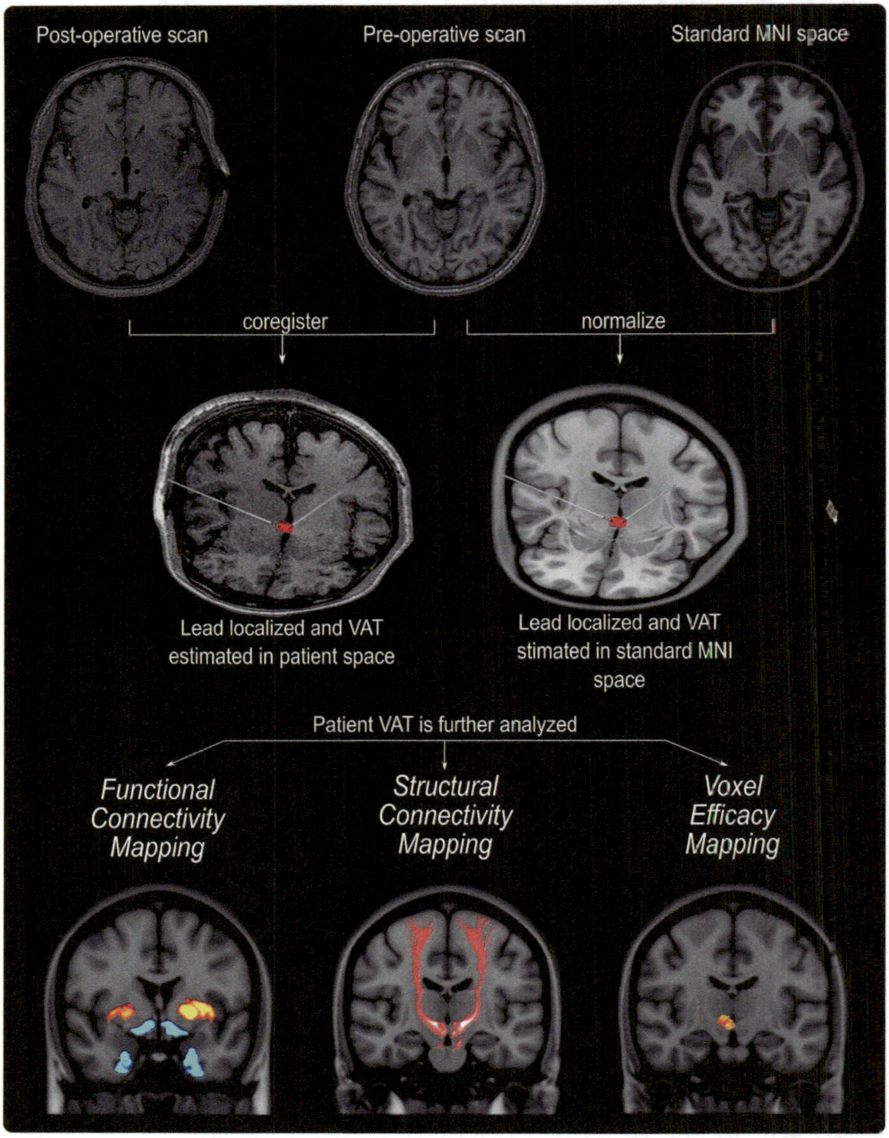

Fig. 6.2 Outline of the different processing steps necessary for electrode localisation using Magnetic Resonance Imaging (MRI). After localisation, modelling can be used to estimate the Volume of Activated Tissue (VAT) and possible further analysis can be performed to investigate the most efficacious stimulation site and brain wide networks associated with clinical outcome. *MNI* Montreal Neurological Institute, *VAT* Volume of Activated Tissue

Volume of Tissue Activated -VTA), the theoretical region where electrical stimulation is conceptualised to elicit additional action potentials [43]. A number of different models with varying complexity have been proposed [16, 18, 19, 44–46]. These allow for the fast and reliable estimation of the anatomical regions within each patient that are affected by the electrical stimulation (Fig. 6.2). Using the estimated VATs of a cohort of patients one can then create voxel-wise efficacy maps of larger regions. Voxel-wise efficacy maps illustrate the spatial pattern and extent associated with beneficial stimulation. These maps provide insight beyond mapping of an ideal target or 'sweet spot' [5–7, 20].

Overall, precise lead localisation and stimulation modelling provide critical input for subsequent DBS programming, suggesting an optimal contact to be used and offering insight into potentially beneficial stimulation parameters. Using the precise lead localisation and observed phenomena occurring intraoperatively or during subsequent programming sessions, one might also use this data, similar to the use of direct cortical stimulation [47–50], to identify the neural substrate of other phenomena [51, 52]

MNI Space and Investigating Potential Mechanisms of DBS

No two human brains are identical, and this variability poses a challenge when comparing findings between patients and when communicating the results of analyses. A common reference space is essential when combining data from larger patient cohorts, and while creating a cohort specific common space is feasible, the use of the Montreal Neurological Institute (MNI) common reference brain space—short 'MNI space' [53–56]—has been established since the 1990s. The MNI space is the common template space for group analyses as well as the reference space to report study findings [57]. Using MNI space also allows for the use of a large number of publicly available brain atlases enabling for example the comparison of study results with meta analyses generated from large numbers of previously reported functional MRI studies [58, 59], or the comparison of findings to detailed human high resolution histology atlases [60] or to patterns of whole brain normative spatial gene expression data [61–63], among others. These atlases enable additional insights to be gleaned into the possible underlying mechanisms of DBS.

Connectomics to Investigate Brain Networks of DBS

Since the brain is a complex network, DBS modulates not only local brain structures but also distributed brain networks [1]. Registering to MNI space allows for the use of normative structural and functional connectomic data to investigate these brain wide networks, while acquiring specialised MRI sequences before surgery makes the analysis of patient-specific connections possible. The term 'connectome' originates from mathematical network models and is used to describe the brain as a network consisting of nodes (anatomical regions) and their connections (structural or functional) [64, 65]. Structural connectomics involves the use of diffusion-weighted MRI (dMRI) that can be employed to estimate structural connectivity, i.e., the white matter connections, between brain regions. dMRI is based on the directionality and anisotropy of water diffusion in each voxel. Functional connectomics makes use of resting-state functional MRI (rsfMRI) to measure the relationship between brain regions based on the covariance of low-frequency blood oxygen level-dependent (BOLD) signal oscillation. Higher covariance indicates that two regions are more related, more functionally connected, based on their functional MRI signal. Multiple studies over the last years have shown that neurological and psychiatric symptoms can be mapped to distributed brain networks using functional and structural connectomics [14, 17, 51, 52, 66–73].

Multiple structural connectomes have been made openly available and are often based on publicly available data. Some were created from dMRI data of healthy individuals, such as the Human Connectome Project (HCP) [74, 75], while others have made use of dMRI data from patients to create a disease-specific connectome, for example the Parkinson's Progression Markers Initiative (PPMI) [76]. Most structural connectomes, both healthy and disease-specific, incorporate data of less than 100 subjects or patients; however, both larger structural [5, 77] and functional connectome created using data of about 1000 healthy subjects have been utilised [5, 14, 52]. One particularly commonly used functional connectome is derived from Brain Genomics Superstruct Project (GSP) [78, 79] data using a 1000-subject, healthy control rsfMRI dataset. Some recent work has made use of smaller disease-specific functional connectomes created using rsfMRI data of patients [52, 80]. The use of disease-specific normative connectomes compared to connectomes derived from healthy participants has some advantages and disadvantages. There are likely differences between the brains of patients with a given neuropsychiatric or neurological disease and healthy subjects [81] and these would not be reflected in healthy normative connectomes [81, 82]. On the other hand, both HCP and GSP data were acquired with specialised MRI hardware offering high fidelity and superior signal-to-noise ratio [83, 84]. Also, some of the healthy connectomes mentioned above are derived from approximately 1000 subjects and recent work has demonstrated that these larger samples allow for more stable and confident estimation of connectivity [85].

Both normative structural and functional connectomics have some limitations that should be considered when designing and interpreting the results of such analyses. It has been shown that brain connections identified by dMRI are partially anatomically incorrect [86, 87] and tend to be biassed towards long, highly myelinated tracts while underestimating short or thin bundles [88, 89]. The MRI signals used for functional connectivity analyses (i.e. BOLD) may be contaminated by other sources of noise [90, 91], are subject to changes depending on patient characteristics (e.g. ageing processes will alter the neurovascular coupling process and result in altered BOLD signal) [92, 93], and may not capture brain activity in higher frequency ranges. Although these limitations apply to both normative and disease-specific connectomes, analyses based on dMRI and rsfMRI are still the only means of investigating structural and functional connectivity in humans in vivo [94]. Moreover, functional and structural connectomics have proven externally applicable by successfully corroborating symptom-associated lesions with efficacious neuromodulation targets. These techniques have been successfully applied to identify the common underlying brain networks implicated in particular symptoms and diseases [67, 68, 70].

Summary and Conclusion

In the past couple of decades there has been an exponential increase in the use of DBS for several distinct clinical indications, along with the interest of investigating lead localisation, modelling of volume of activated tissue, and whole brain connectomics to understand the underlying neurobiological mechanisms of action of DBS and to further optimise DBS treatment. As outlined, MRI is an essential tool for this endeavour. It can be used to localise DBS in individual patients with high accuracy, offering the particular advantage of precise target confirmation especially when employing some of the newly developed specialised sequences that offer enhanced tissue contrast in the anatomical region of interest. This information can be used directly to inform clinical treatment plans through identifying the optimal contact and informing the stimulation parameters to be interrogated. Also, once the electrodes are successfully localised, scientists may use advanced modelling of the electrical field induced combined with a number of state-of-the-art imaging analysis tools to investigate the potential underlying mechanisms of action of DBS, the brain network implicated in efficacious treatment as well as determining the ideal target location. MRI and the advanced analysis tools described here have contributed tremendously to our growing understanding of the mechanisms and brain networks involved in symptom alleviation following DBS treatment.

References

1. Lozano AM, Lipsman N, Bergman H, et al. Deep brain stimulation: current challenges and future directions. Nat Rev Neurol. 2019;15:148–60.
2. Lozano AM, Eltahawy H. How does DBS work? Suppl Clin Neurophysiol. 2004;57:733–6.
3. Horn A, Li N, Dembek TA, et al. Lead-DBS v2: towards a comprehensive pipeline for deep brain stimulation imaging. NeuroImage. 2019;184:293–316.
4. Bot M, Schuurman PR, Odekerken VJJ, Verhagen R, Contarino FM, De Bie RMA, van den Munckhof P. Deep brain stimulation for Parkinson's disease: defining the optimal location within the subthalamic nucleus. J Neurol Neurosurg Psychiatry. 2018 89:493–8.
5. Elias GJB, Boutet A, Joel SE, et al. Probabilistic mapping of deep brain stimulation: insights from 15 years of therapy. Ann Neurol. 2020; https://doi.org/10.1002/ana.25975.
6. Boutet A, Germann J, Gwun D, et al. Sign-specific stimulation "hot" and "cold" spots in Parkinson's disease validated with machine learning. Brain Commun 2021;3:fcab027.

7. Dembek TA, Roediger J, Horn A, et al. Probabilistic sweet spots predict motor outcome for deep brain stimulation in Parkinson disease. Ann Neurol. 2019;86:527–38.
8. Petry-Schmelzer JN, Krause M, Dembek TA, et al. Non-motor outcomes depend on location of neurostimulation in Parkinson's disease. Brain. 2019;142:3592–604.
9. Dembek TA, Baldermann C, Petry-Schmelzer J-N, Jergas H, Treuer H, Visser-Vandewalle V, Dafsari HS, Barbe MT. Sweetspot mapping in deep brain stimulation: strengths and limitations of current approaches. Neurology. 2020; https://doi.org/10.1101/2020.09.08.20190223.
10. Geng X, Xu X, Horn A, Li N, Ling Z, Brown P, Wang S. Intra-operative characterisation of subthalamic oscillations in Parkinson's disease. Clin Neurophysiol. 2018;129:1001–10.
11. Neumann W-J, Horn A, Ewert S, Huebl J, Brücke C, Slentz C, Schneider G-H, Kühn AA. A localized pallidal physiomarker in cervical dystonia. Ann Neurol. 2017;82:912–24.
12. Milosevic L, Kalia SK, Hodaie M, Lozano AM, Popovic MR, Hutchison WD, Lankarany M. A theoretical framework for the site-specific and frequency-dependent neuronal effects of deep brain stimulation. Brain Stimul. 2021; https://doi.org/10.1016/j.brs.2021.04.022.
13. Germann J, Boutet A, Elias GJB, Gouveia FV, Loh A, Giacobbe P, Bhat V, Kucharczyk W, Lozano AM. Brain structures and networks underlying treatment response to deep brain stimulation targeting the inferior thalamic peduncle in obsessive-compulsive disorder. Stereotact Funct Neurosurg. 2022:1–8.
14. Li N, Hollunder B, Baldermann JC, et al. A unified functional network target for deep brain stimulation in obsessive-compulsive disorder. Biol Psychiatry. 2021; https://doi.org/10.1016/j.biopsych.2021.04.006.
15. Vetkas A, Germann J, Elias G, et al. Identifying the neural network for neuromodulation in epilepsy through connectomics and graphs. Brain Commun. 2022;4:fcac092.
16. Horn A, Reich M, Vorwerk J, et al. Connectivity predicts deep brain stimulation outcome in Parkinson disease. Ann Neurol. 2017;82:67–78.
17. Elias GJB, Germann J, Boutet A, et al. Structuro-functional surrogates of response to subcallosal cingulate deep brain stimulation for depression. Brain. 2021; https://doi.org/10.1093/brain/awab284.
18. Butson CR, McIntyre CC. Current steering to control the volume of tissue activated during deep brain stimulation. Brain Stimul. 2008;1:7–15.
19. Dembek TA, Barbe MT, Åström M, Hoevels M, Visser-Vandewalle V, Fink GR, Timmermann L. Probabilistic mapping of deep brain stimulation effects in essential tremor. Neuroimage Clin. 2017;13:164–73.
20. Eisenstein SA, Koller JM, Black KD, et al. Functional anatomy of subthalamic nucleus stimulation in Parkinson disease. Ann Neurol. 2014;76:279–95.
21. Treu S, Strange B, Oxenford S, Neumann W-J, Kühn A, Li N, Horn A. Deep brain stimulation: imaging on a group level. NeuroImage. 2020;219:117018.
22. Montgomery EB Jr. Validation of CT-MRI fusion for intraoperative assessment of stereotactic accuracy in DBS surgery. Mov Disord. 2015;30:439.
23. Pinsker MO, Herzog J, Falk D, Volkmann J, Deuschl G, Mehdorn M. Accuracy and distortion of deep brain stimulation electrodes on postoperative MRI and CT. Zentralbl Neurochir. 2008;69:144–7.
24. Kremer NI, Oterdoom DLM, van Laar PJ, Piña-Fuentes D, van Laar T, Drost G, van Hulzen ALJ, van Dijk JMC. Accuracy of intraoperative computed tomography in deep brain stimulation-a prospective noninferiority study. Neuromodulation. 2019;22:472–7.
25. Matias CM, Frizon LA, Asfahan F, Uribe JD, Machado AG. Brain shift and pneumocephalus assessment during frame-based deep brain stimulation implantation with intraoperative magnetic resonance imaging. Oper Neurosurg. 2018;14:668–74.
26. Liu X, Zhang J, Fu K, Gong R, Chen J, Zhang J. Microelectrode recording-guided versus intraoperative magnetic resonance imaging-guided subthalamic nucleus deep brain stimulation surgery for Parkinson disease: a 1-year follow-up study. World Neurosurg. 2017;107:900–5.
27. Pinto S, Le Bas J-F, Castana L, Krack P, Pollak P, Benabid A-L. Comparison of two techniques to postoperatively localize the electrode contacts used for subthalamic nucleus stimulation. Oper Neurosurg. 2007;60:285–94.

28. Hyam JA, Akram H, Foltynie T, Limousin P, Hariz M, Zrinzo L. What you see is what you get: Lead location within deep brain structures is accurately depicted by stereotactic magnetic resonance imaging. Oper Neurosurg. 2015;11:412.
29. Miyagi Y, Shima F, Sasaki T. Brain shift: an error factor during implantation of deep brain stimulation electrodes. J Neurosurg. 2007;107:989–97.
30. Elias WJ, Fu K-M, Frysinger RC. Cortical and subcortical brain shift during stereotactic procedures. J Neurosurg. 2007;107:983–8.
31. Pollo C, Vingerhoets F, Pralong E, Ghika J, Maeder P, Meuli R, Thiran J-P, Villemure J-G. Localization of electrodes in the subthalamic nucleus on magnetic resonance imaging. J Neurosurg. 2007;106:36–44.
32. Lee JY, Kim JW, Lee J-Y, Lim YH, Kim C, Kim DG, Jeon BS, Paek SH. Is MRI a reliable tool to locate the electrode after deep brain stimulation surgery? Comparison study of CT and MRI for the localization of electrodes after DBS. Acta Neurochir. 2010;152:2029–36.
33. Yelnik J, Damier P, Demeret S, et al. Localization of stimulating electrodes in patients with Parkinson disease by using a three-dimensional atlas-magnetic resonance imaging coregistration method. J Neurosurg. 2003;99:89–99.
34. Hamid NA, Mitchell RD, Mocroft P, Westby GWM, Milner J, Pall H. Targeting the subthalamic nucleus for deep brain stimulation: technical approach and fusion of pre- and postoperative MR images to define accuracy of lead placement. J Neurol Neurosurg Psychiatry. 2005;76:409–14.
35. He C, Zhang F, Li L, Jiang C, Li L. Measurement of lead localization accuracy based on magnetic resonance imaging. Front Neurosci. 2021;15:632822.
36. Boutet A, Chow CT, Narang K, et al. Improving safety of MRI in patients with deep brain stimulation devices. Radiology. 2020;296:250–62.
37. Boutet A, Rashid T, Hancu I, et al. Functional MRI safety and artifacts during deep brain stimulation: experience in 102 patients. Radiology. 2019;293:174–83.
38. Horn A. The impact of modern-day neuroimaging on the field of deep brain stimulation. Curr Opin Neurol. 2019;32:511–20.
39. Boutet A, Loh A, Chow CT, et al. A literature review of magnetic resonance imaging sequence advancements in visualizing functional neurosurgery targets. J Neurosurg. 2021;1:1–14.
40. Neudorfer C, Kroneberg D, Al-Fatly B, et al. Personalizing deep brain stimulation using advanced imaging sequences. Ann Neurol. 2022; https://doi.org/10.1002/ana.26326.
41. Middlebrooks EH, Tipton P, Okromelidze L, Greco E, Mendez JA, Uitti R, Grewal SS. Deep brain stimulation for tremor: direct targeting of a novel imaging biomarker. Ann Neurol. 2022; https://doi.org/10.1002/ana.26422.
42. Al Awadhi A, Tyrand R, Horn A, Kibleur A, Vincentini J, Zacharia A, Burkhard PR, Momjian S, Boëx C. Electrophysiological confrontation of Lead-DBS-based electrode localizations in patients with Parkinson's disease undergoing deep brain stimulation. NeuroImage: Clin. 2022;34:102971.
43. McIntyre CC, Grill WM. Extracellular stimulation of central neurons: influence of stimulus waveform and frequency on neuronal output. J Neurophysiol. 2002;88:1592–604.
44. Kuncel AM, Cooper SE, Grill WM. A method to estimate the spatial extent of activation in thalamic deep brain stimulation. Clin Neurophysiol. 2008;119:2148–58.
45. Astrom M, Diczfalusy E, Martens H, Wardell K. Relationship between neural activation and electric field distribution during deep brain stimulation. IEEE Trans Biomed Eng. 2015;62:664–72.
46. Mädler B, Coenen VA. Explaining clinical effects of deep brain stimulation through simplified target-specific modeling of the volume of activated tissue. Am J Neuroradiol. 2012;33:1072–80.
47. Lu J, Zhao Z, Zhang J, Wu B, Zhu Y, Chang EF, Wu J, Duffau H, Berger MS. Functional maps of direct electrical stimulation-induced speech arrest and anomia: a multicentre retrospective study. Brain. 2021;144:2541–53.
48. Penfield W, Boldrey E. Somatic motor and sensory representation in the cerebral cortex of man as studied by electrical stimulation. Brain. 1937;60:389–443.

49. Penfield W, Rasmussen T. The cerebral cortex of man: a clinical study of localization of function. Macmillan; 1950.
50. Roux F-E, Djidjeli I, Durand J-B. Functional architecture of the somatosensory homunculus detected by electrostimulation. J Physiol. 2018;596:941–56.
51. Neudorfer C, Elias GJB, Jakobs M, et al. Mapping autonomic, mood and cognitive effects of hypothalamic region deep brain stimulation. Brain. 2021;144:2837–51.
52. Germann J, Elias GJB, Boutet A, et al. Brain structures and networks responsible for stimulation-induced memory flashbacks during forniceal deep brain stimulation for Alzheimer's disease. Alzheimers Dement. 2021;17:777–87.
53. Fonov VS, Evans AC, McKinstry RC, Almli CR, Collins DL. Unbiased nonlinear average age-appropriate brain templates from birth to adulthood. NeuroImage. 2009;47:S102.
54. Talairach J, Tournoux P. Co-planar stereotaxic atlas of the human brain. 3-dimensional proportional system: an approach to imaging. 1988. Stuttgart, New York: Georg Thieme Verlag; 1988. Thieme Medical Publishers, Inc…
55. Mazziotta JC, Toga AW, Evans A, Fox P, Lancaster J. A probabilistic atlas of the human brain: theory and rationale for its development. NeuroImage. 1995;2:89–101.
56. Mazziotta J, Toga A, Evans A, et al. A probabilistic atlas and reference system for the human brain: international consortium for brain mapping (ICBM). Philos Trans R Soc Lond Ser B Biol Sci. 2001;356:1293–322.
57. Brett M, Johnsrude IS, Owen AM. The problem of functional localization in the human brain. Nat Rev Neurosci. 2002;3:243–9.
58. Geniesse C, Chowdhury S, Saggar M. NeuMapper: a scalable computational framework for multiscale exploration of the brain's dynamical organization. Netw Neurosci. 2022;6:467–98.
59. Yarkoni T, Poldrack RA, Nichols TE, Van Essen DC, Wager TD. Large-scale automated synthesis of human functional neuroimaging data. Nat Methods. 2011;8:665–70.
60. Amunts K, Lepage C, Borgeat L, et al. BigBrain: an ultrahigh-resolution 3D human brain model. Science. 2013;340:1472–5.
61. Shen EH, Overly CC, Jones AR. The Allen human brain atlas: comprehensive gene expression mapping of the human brain. Trends Neurosci. 2012;35:711–4.
62. Jones AR, Overly CC, Sunkin SM. The Allen brain atlas: 5 years and beyond. Nat Rev Neurosci. 2009;10:821–8.
63. Hawrylycz MJ, Lein ES, Guillozet-Bongaarts AL, et al. An anatomically comprehensive atlas of the adult human brain transcriptome. Nature. 2012;489:391–9.
64. van den Heuvel MP, Sporns O. A cross-disorder connectome landscape of brain dysconnectivity. Nat Rev Neurosci. 2019;20:435–46.
65. Sporns O, Tononi G, Kötter R. The human connectome: a structural description of the human brain. PLoS Comput Biol. 2005;1:0245–51.
66. Boutet A, Madhavan R, Elias GJB, et al. Predicting optimal deep brain stimulation parameters for Parkinson's disease using functional MRI and machine learning. Nat Commun. 2021;12:3043.
67. Germann J, Elias GJB, Neudorfer C, et al. Potential optimization of focused ultrasound capsulotomy for obsessive compulsive disorder. Brain. 2021; https://doi.org/10.1093/brain/awab232.
68. Siddiqi SH, Schaper FLWVJ, Horn A, et al. Brain stimulation and brain lesions converge on common causal circuits in neuropsychiatric disease. Nat Hum Behav. 2021; https://doi.org/10.1038/s41562-021-01161-1.
69. Fox MD. Mapping symptoms to brain networks with the human connectome. N Engl J Med. 2018;379:2237–45.
70. Fox MD, Buckner RL, Liu H, Chakravarty MM, Lozano AM, Pascual-Leone A. Resting-state networks link invasive and noninvasive brain stimulation across diverse psychiatric and neurological diseases. Proc Natl Acad Sci U S A. 2014;111:E4367–75.
71. Cohen AL, Ferguson MA, Fox MD. Lesion network mapping predicts post-stroke behavioural deficits and improves localization. Brain. 2021; https://doi.org/10.1093/brain/awab002.

72. Darby RR, Joutsa J, Fox MD. Network localization of heterogeneous neuroimaging findings. Brain. 2019;142:70–9.
73. Corp DT, Joutsa J, Darby RR, et al. Network localization of cervical dystonia based on causal brain lesions. Brain. 2019;142:1660–74.
74. Glasser MF, Sotiropoulos SN, Wilson JA, et al. The minimal preprocessing pipelines for the human connectome project. NeuroImage. 2013;80:105–24.
75. Glasser MF, Smith SM, Marcus DS, et al. The human connectome Project's neuroimaging approach. Nat Neurosci. 2016;19:1175–87.
76. The Parkinson Progression Marker Initiative (PPMI). Prog Neurobiol. 2011;95:629–35.
77. Li N, Baldermann JC, Kibleur A, et al. A unified connectomic target for deep brain stimulation in obsessive-compulsive disorder. Nat Commun. 2020;11:3364.
78. Holmes AJ, Hollinshead MO, O'Keefe TM, et al. Brain genomics Superstruct project initial data release with structural, functional, and behavioral measures. Sci Data. 2015;2:150031.
79. Yeo BTT, Krienen FM, Sepulcre J, et al. The organization of the human cerebral cortex estimated by intrinsic functional connectivity. J Neurophysiol. 2011;106:1125–65.
80. Loh A, Boutet A, Germann J, et al. A functional connectome of Parkinson's disease patients prior to deep brain stimulation: a tool for disease-specific connectivity analyses. Front Neurosci. 2022; https://doi.org/10.3389/fnins.2022.804125.
81. Bassett DS, Bullmore ET. Human brain networks in health and disease. Curr Opin Neurol. 2009;22:340–7.
82. Klobušiaková P, Mareček R, Fousek J, Výtvarová E, Rektorová I. Connectivity between brain networks dynamically reflects cognitive status of Parkinson's disease: a longitudinal study. J Alzheimers Dis. 2019;67:971–84.
83. Setsompop K, Kimmlingen R, Eberlein E, et al. Pushing the limits of in vivo diffusion MRI for the human connectome project. NeuroImage. 2013;80:220–33.
84. Elam JS, Glasser MF, Harms MP, et al. The human connectome project: a retrospective. NeuroImage. 2021:118543.
85. Cohen AL, Fox MD. Reply: the influence of sample size and arbitrary statistical thresholds in lesion-network mapping. Brain. 2020; https://doi.org/10.1093/brain/awaa095.
86. Maier-Hein KH, Neher PF, Houde J-C, et al. The challenge of mapping the human connectome based on diffusion tractography. Nat Commun. 2017;8:1349.
87. Thomas C, Ye FQ, Irfanoglu MO, Modi P, Saleem KS, Leopold DA, Pierpaoli C. Anatomical accuracy of brain connections derived from diffusion MRI tractography is inherently limited. Proc Natl Acad Sci U S A. 2014;111:16574–9.
88. Zhang Y, Zhang J, Oishi K, et al. Atlas-guided tract reconstruction for automated and comprehensive examination of the white matter anatomy. NeuroImage. 2010;52:1289–301.
89. Alho EJL, Alho ATDL, Horn A, Martin M d GM, Edlow BL, Fiscal B, Nagy J, Fonoff ET, Hamani C, Heinsen H. The Ansa Subthalamica: a neglected Fiber tract. Mov Disord. 2020;35:75–80.
90. Murphy K, Fox MD. Towards a consensus regarding global signal regression for resting state functional connectivity MRI. NeuroImage. 2017;154:169–73.
91. Fox MD, Raichle ME. Spontaneous fluctuations in brain activity observed with functional magnetic resonance imaging. Nat Rev Neurosci. 2007;8:700–11.
92. Tsvetanov KA, Henson RNA, Tyler LK, Davis SW, Shafto MA, Taylor JR, Williams N, Cam-Can RJB. The effect of ageing on fMRI: correction for the confounding effects of vascular reactivity evaluated by joint fMRI and MEG in 335 adults. Hum Brain Mapp. 2015;36:2248–69.
93. Girouard H, Iadecola C. Neurovascular coupling in the normal brain and in hypertension, stroke, and Alzheimer disease. J Appl Physiol. 2006;100:328–35.
94. Conturo TE, Lori NF, Cull TS, Akbudak E, Snyder AZ, Shimony JS, McKinstry RC, Burton H, Raichle ME. Tracking neuronal fiber pathways in the living human brain. Proc Natl Acad Sci U S A. 1999;96:10422–7.

7 Acquiring Functional Magnetic Resonance Imaging in Patients Treated with Deep Brain Stimulation

Dave Gwun, Aaron Loh, Artur Vetkas, Alexandre Boutet, Mojgan Hodaie, Suneil K. Kalia, Alfonso Fasano, and Andres M. Lozano

Dave Gwun, Aaron Loh and Artur Vetkas contributed equally to this work

D. Gwun (✉) · A. Loh · A. Vetkas
Division of Neurosurgery, University Health Network and University of Toronto, Toronto, ON, Canada

A. Boutet
Division of Neurosurgery, University Health Network and University of Toronto, Toronto, ON, Canada

Joint Department of Medical Imaging, University of Toronto, Toronto, ON, Canada
e-mail: alexandre.boutet@mail.utoronto.ca

M. Hodaie · A. M. Lozano
Division of Neurosurgery, University Health Network and University of Toronto, Toronto, ON, Canada

Krembil Research Institute, Toronto, ON, Canada
e-mail: mojgan.hodaie@uhn.ca; lozano@uhnresearch.ca

S. K. Kalia
Division of Neurosurgery, University Health Network and University of Toronto, Toronto, ON, Canada

Krembil Research Institute, Toronto, ON, Canada

Center for Advancing Neurotechnological Innovation to Application (CRANIA), Toronto, ON, Canada
e-mail: Suneil.Kalia@uhn.ca

A. Fasano
Krembil Research Institute, Toronto, ON, Canada

Center for Advancing Neurotechnological Innovation to Application (CRANIA), Toronto, ON, Canada

A. Boutet, A. M. Lozano (eds.), *Magnetic Resonance Imaging in Deep Brain Stimulation*, https://doi.org/10.1007/978-3-031-16348-7_7

Edmond J. Safra Program in Parkinson's Disease and Morton and Gloria Shulman Movement Disorders Clinic, Toronto Western Hospital and Division of Neurology, UHN, Division of Neurology, University of Toronto, Toronto, ON, Canada

GE Global Research Center, Niskayuna, NY, USA
e-mail: alfonso.fasano@uhn.ca

Introduction

Deep brain stimulation (DBS) is a reversible and adjustable neurosurgical treatment that involves electrically stimulating brain structures through stereotactically implanted electrodes [1–4]. Since its inception in the early 1960s, over 200,000 patients have been treated with DBS [4]. While DBS is most commonly used to alleviate the motor symptoms of Parkinson's disease (PD) and essential tremor (ET), it is also a promising treatment for several refractory neurological and psychiatric conditions, including obsessive-compulsive disorder (OCD), epilepsy, Tourette Syndrome (TS), Alzheimer's disease, and chronic pain [4]. Despite its growing utilization, the mechanisms of DBS remain largely unknown. Additionally, DBS patient selection and programming are time and resource intensive and largely dependent on empirical clinical experience and trial-and-error [4]. This highlights the need for research tools that can enhance our understanding of DBS and aberrant neural networks behind neuropsychiatric disorders, as well as biomarkers that can optimize DBS patient selection, targeting, and programming.

Functional neuroimaging modalities, such as positron emission tomography (PET), single-photon emission computed tomography (SPECT), magnetoencephalography (MEG), and functional magnetic resonance imaging (fMRI), offer insights into local and global changes in brain activity and connectivity. These modalities can be used to interrogate neural responses to DBS and investigate the function of neural circuits with respect to disease, cognition, and behavior [5–7]. fMRI is unique among these imaging modalities as it is readily available at most centers and does not involve radiation or the administration of exogenous contrast [8]. fMRI can measure blood-oxygen-level-dependent (BOLD) signals, a type of "endogenous contrast," to detect changes in brain metabolism [9, 10]. Additionally, fMRI provides a good balance between spatial and temporal resolution compared to other modalities [8]. Despite these advantages, the use of fMRI in DBS patients has been limited by safety guidelines, namely the risk of electrode heating during fMRI acquisition [8, 11–13]. Technical challenges, such as loss of signal from susceptibility artifacts related to DBS hardware, may have further delayed the widespread application of fMRI in DBS patients [8, 11–13].

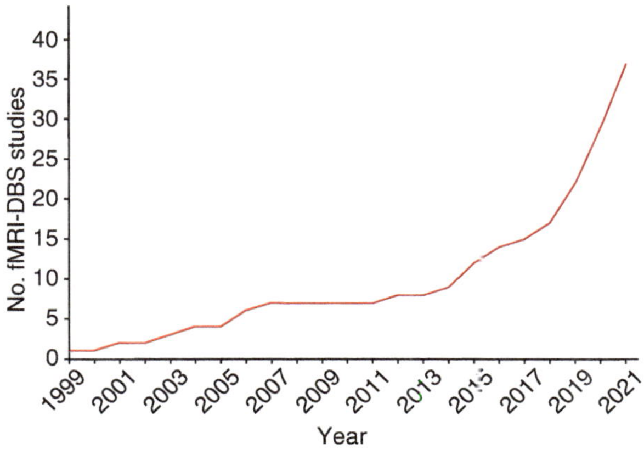

Fig. 7.1 The cumulative number of fMRI-DBS studies from 1999 to 2021

Consequently, studies have often investigated the effects of DBS on brain networks by relying on publicly available functional connectivity templates acquired from large cohorts of healthy volunteers, also called "normative connectome" [14–17]. Such studies estimate the connectivity between a given brain region and the stimulation location in a normative (i.e., averaged "normal") brain and are herein referred to as normative fMRI studies. In contrast, studies that acquire fMRI from patients after DBS surgery with stimulation on and off are referred to as "patient-specific fMRI studies" [18–21]. While normative fMRI studies have the advantage of using large, high-quality fMRI datasets, they are limited by the fact that they might not reflect patient- or disease-specific connectivity. Furthermore, normative connectome studies cannot assess brain network responses to DBS in a causal manner [16]. Conversely, patient-specific fMRI is acquired in DBS patients and can directly assess the effects of stimulation on the brain [16, 21]. The information gathered from patient-specific fMRI studies can thus be used to obtain valuable insights into the mechanisms of DBS, provide biomarkers associated with therapeutic outcomes, and produce vast theoretical knowledge about the neurological conditions associated with aberrant neural networks [2, 16, 22].

To date, 37 patient-specific fMRI-DBS studies have been published, reporting findings from over 400 patients with various DBS indications and targets. The number of studies that applied fMRI in DBS patients has steadily increased over the last three years (Fig. 7.1). This increase may be attributable to recent advances in fMRI acquisition, safety, and analyses methods which have improved the quality and reliability of findings. Here, we describe challenges in acquiring fMRI in DBS patients, experimental design paradigms, and analyses methods employed by fMRI-DBS studies and summarize the main characteristics and findings of these studies, including the effect of DBS on various disorders and neural networks.

Challenges Associated with Acquiring fMRI in DBS Patients

Safety considerations associated with scanning DBS patients with MRI include potential injuries caused by heating of electrode tips, induced currents, implantable pulse generator dysfunction, and mechanical forces, of which electrode heating is

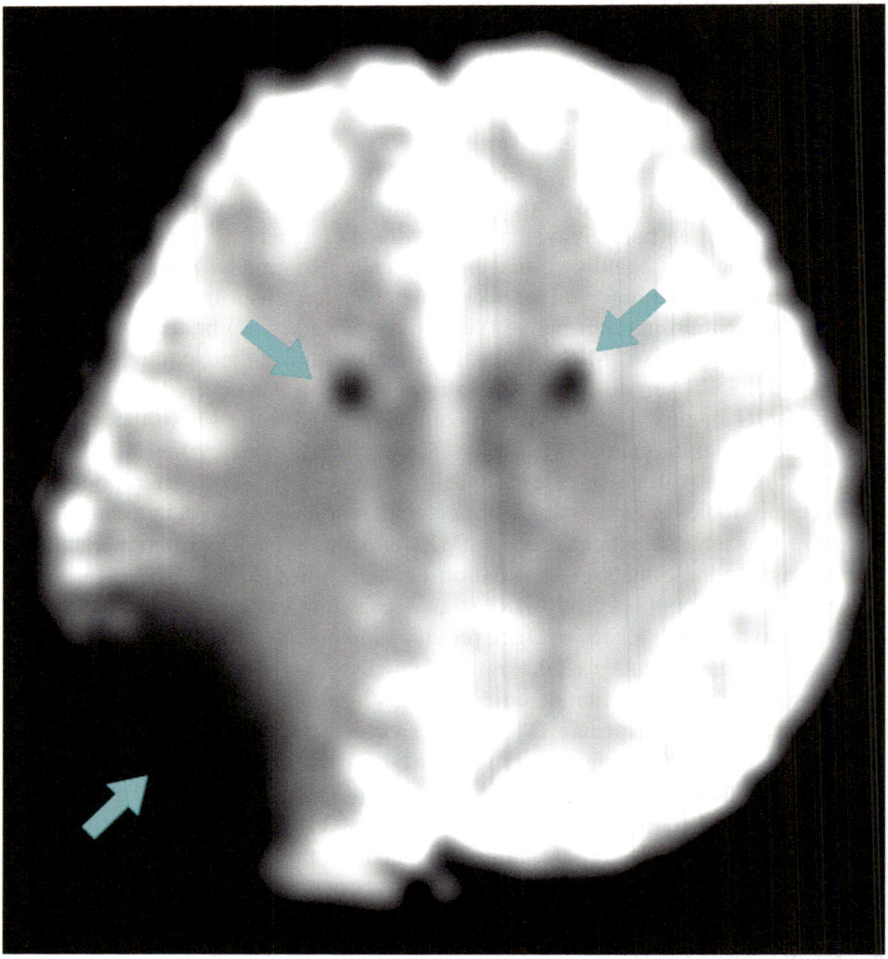

Fig. 7.2 Metal susceptibility artifact associated with DBS hardware. Axial slices of gradient-recalled echo-echo planar imaging acquired from a patient treated with DBS. Blue arrows indicate the metal susceptibility artifact produced by the DBS coil and electrode

the primary concern [11]. These have been addressed by early fMRI-DBS studies—and subsequent safety and phantom studies—which confirmed that 1.5 T and 3 T MRI acquisitions are safe in patients with DBS under specific scanning conditions (i.e., low specific absorption rate, certain geometry of DBS hardware in relation to the scanner) and with thorough prior safety testing [12, 23]. However, it should be emphasized that guidelines for scanning vary for each DBS manufacturer.

fMRI in patients with DBS is additionally limited by technical challenges, including the susceptibility artifact from the DBS electrode and subgaleal wires (Fig. 7.2) [13]. While susceptibility artifact leads to signal loss around the subcortical stimulation targets and cortical regions adjacent to the coil wire (e.g., primary motor cortex—M1), it should be highlighted that the artifacts only affect a small portion of the brain (mean electrode contact artifact diameter = 9.3 mm and coil artifact accounts for 1.9–2.1% of the whole-brain volume) [13]. Previous DBS-fMRI studies have accounted for these artifacts by performing unilateral stimulation [22, 24–26], segmenting and masking areas of signal loss to exclude affected regions from the analysis [27–34], or assessing brain regions with significant signal loss (i.e., subthalamic nucleus) as "hidden nodes" [35, 36]. Of note, a recent study was able to extract useful BOLD signal near the electrode such as brain areas within the volume of tissue activated despite the presence of the metal artifact [37].

fMRI Study Results

The study characteristics including the sample size, DBS indication and target, and experimental design of the 37 patient-specific fMRI-DBS studies are summarized in Table 7.1. Apart from a few recent studies, fMRI-DBS studies include small sample sizes (mean = 13 ± 13, median = 10, IQR = 11). It should be noted that interpreting and comparing fMRI findings should be done with caution as BOLD signal responses and network connectivity can change dramatically based on many variables including the study cohort, fMRI experimental design and scanning conditions, stimulation parameters, analysis methods, or a combination of these factors.

fMRI Acquisition, Experimental Design Paradigms and Analysis

Depending on a study's research question and hypothesis, the fMRI acquisition and experimental design can vary significantly between studies. For clarity, this review categorizes fMRI experimental designs into three broad paradigms: (1) resting-state, (2) task-based, and (3) cycling-stimulation (Fig. 7.3).

As the name suggests, resting-state fMRI (rs-fMRI) design involves scanning subjects at rest with their eyes open or closed and where the experimental or stimulation conditions remain constant throughout the duration of the scan. The decision to instruct participants to open or close their eyes depends on the research question and hypothesis; however, both conditions present comparable results [10]. Conversely, in task-based fMRI, participants perform tasks (e.g., finger-tapping) specifically designed to induce brain changes while being scanned. fMRI-DBS

Table 7.1 Summary of fMRI-DBS study characteristics and reported brain areas

First author (yr) (ref)	Disease (n)	Target	Post-op to scan	MRI	Design	Task	Comparators	Reported brain areas
Rezai et al. (1999)[a] [23]	ET (2)	VIM	NS	1.5 T Siemens	cs-fMRI	NA	DBS ON/OFF	SI, SII, Th, In, CC
Gibson et al. (2016) [38]	ET (10)	VIM	Intra-op; 1 week	1.5 T GE	cs-fMRI	NA	DBS ON/OFF	SMC, Th, Cer, SMA, BS, IFG
Awad et al. (2020) [29]	ET (16)	cZI	≥ 11 months	1.5 T Philips	cs-fMRI; tb-fMRI	Postural holding; pointing; resting	DBS ON/OFF x task	SMC, SMA, Cer, PMC
Jech et al. (2001) [39]	PD (4)	STN (3); VIM (1)	NS	1.5 T Siemens	cs-fMRI	NA	DBS ON/OFF	GPi, Th, SN, SC, DLPFC LPMC, CN
Stefurak et al. (2003) [40]	PD w/ depression (1)	STN	1 week	1.5 T GE	cs-fMRI	NA	DBS ON/OFF	PMC, MC, Th, Pu, SMC, PFC, ACC
Hesselmann et al. (2004) [41]	PD (1)	STN	Day of surgery	1.5 T Philips	tb-fMRI	Finger opposition	DBS ON/OFF x task	SMC, Cer
Phillips et al. (2006) [25]	PD (5)	STN	1–2 days	3 T GE	cs-fMRI	NA	DBS ON/OFF	BGe, Pu, Th, Cer, SN
Arantes et al. (2006) [31]	PD (4)	STN	Pre-op; Post-op	1.5 T Siemens	tb-fMRI	Finger-tapping, foot flexion and extension, foot rotation, tongue movement	DBS ON/OFF x Task Modality x Task Complexity x Laterality	NS
Kahan et al. (2012) [32]	PD (10)	STN	≥ 8 months	1.5 T Siemens	tb-fMRI	Joystick movement	DBS ON/OFF x task x laterality	TCC
Kahan et al. (2014) [35]	PD (12)	STN	≥ 8 months	1.5 T Siemens	rs-fMRI; tb fMRI	Joystick movement	DBS ON/OFF x task x laterality	CSC, TCC, STC, SSC, STC, CSTC

Holiga et al. (2015) [34]	PD (13)	STN	Day of surgery 1–3 days	1.5 T GE	rs-fMRI	NA	DBS ON/OFF x Pre-/Post-op	PMC
Knight et al. (2015) [42]	PD (10)	STN	Intra-op	1.5 T Siemens	cs-fMRI	NA	DBS ON/OFF x Awake/General anesthesia states	PM, PMC, SMA, PPN, CC, In
Saenger et al. (2017) [27]	PD (10); HC (49)	STN	≥ 6 months	1.5 T Siemens	rs-fMRI	NA	DBS ON/OFF x DBS/HC	WBFC
Mueller et al. (2018) [43]	PD (13)	STN	1–3 days	1.5 T Siemens	rs-fMRI	NA	DBS ON/OFF x Pre-/Post-op	CTCC
Hancu et al. (2019) [26]	PD (13)	STN	≥ 4 months	1.5 & 3 T	cs-fMRI	NA	DBS ON/OFF x Mono−/bipolar settings	NA
Horn et al. (2019) [37]	PD (20); HC (15)	STN	≥ 3 months	1.5 T GE	rs-fMRI	NA	DBS/HC x Electrode placement; Stimulation amplitude	Th, MC, St, Cer, GPe, STN, SMC
DiMarzio et al. (2019) [28]	PD (10); no DBS (15)	STN	NS	1.5 & 3 T Siemens	tb-fMRI	Mechanical pain stimuli	DBS ON/OFF x stimuli	SI, CC
Kahan et al. (2019) [36]	PD (11)	STN	≥ 3 months	1.5 T Siemens	rs-fMRI, tb-fMRI	Joystick movement	DBS ON/OFF x task x Laterality	CSC, TCC, STC
Hanssen et al. (2019) [24]	PD (26)	STN	≥ 3 months	1.5 T Philips	rs-fMRI	NA	DBS ON/OFF	Cer, Pu, PFC
DiMarzio et al. (2020) [33]	PD (23)	STN (15); GPi (8)	NS	1.5 & 3 T GE	cs-fMRI	NA	PD phenotype x (Non-)/Optimal lead placement; TEED; UPDRS-III; 3/1.5 T MRI	Th, GPe, phenotype dependent
DiMarzio et al. (2020) [44]	PD (14)	STN	NS	1.5 & 3 T GE	cs-fMRI	NA	DBS ON/OFF x frequency (optimal±30/60 Hz)	GPe, Cer, Th, SI

(continued)

Table 7.1 (continued)

First author (yr) (ref)	Disease (n)	Target	Post-op to scan	MRI	Design	Task	Comparators	Reported brain areas
Shen et al. (2020) [45]	PD (14)	STN	1 month preop; 1, 3, 6, 12 month	3 T Siemens	cs-fMRI	NA	DBS ON/OFF x DBS frequency x Follow-up time	GP, Th, Cer, M1, Pu, SMA
Mueller et al. (2020) [30]	PD (32)	STN	1–3 days	1.5 T Philips	tb-fMRI	Finger-tapping	DBS ON/OFF x task x L-DOPA ON/OFF	Pu
Gibson et al. (2021) [46]	PD (20)	STN	1 week	1.5 T GE	cs-fMRI	NA	DBS ON/OFF	Cer, Po, Th, PCC, Occ, PCG, Pu, In
Boutet et al. (2021) [22]	PD (67)	STN (62); GPi (5)	≥ 1.4 months	3 T GE	cs-fMRI	NA	DBS ON/OFF x (Non-)/Optimal contacts x (Non-)/Optimal voltage	Th, MC, Cer, iFr, Occ
Zhang et al. (2021) [47]	PD (55)	STN (27); GPi (28)	STN (10 months) GPi (21.3 months)	1.5 T Siemens	rs-fMRI	NA	DBS ON/OFF	TCC, SMCC
Steinhardt et al. (2021) [48]	PD (21)	STN	23.9 months	1.5 T Philips	tb-fMRI	Sweet, savory, or neutral food presentation	DBS ON/OFF x food conditions	IN, SMG, Th, Am, PF
Baker et al. (2007) [49]	OCD (1)	ALIC	2 days	3 T Siemens	cs-fMRI	NA	(Non-)/Optimal contacts x Laterality	Ca, Th, ACC, Cer
Hiss et al. (2015) [50]	OCD (3)	NAc/ALIC	Intra-op	1.5 T Philips	cs-fMRI; tb-fMRI	NA	Disgust stimuli x Frequencies intensity	NAc, ACC, St
Gibson et al. (2016) [51]	OCD (4)	VC/VS	Intra-op	1.5 T GE	cs-fMRI	NA	DBS ON/OFF x (Non-)/Mirth inducing settings	CSTC, Am, VS, Th, ACC
Elias et al. (2021) [52]	AN (9), Depression (6), BD (1)	SCC	1.2–15.7 years	3 T GE	rs-fMRI	N	DBS ON/OFF x (Non-)/optimal settings	dACC, PCC, PCu, IPL
Rezai et al. (1999)[a] [23]	Pain (3)	Vc; PVG	NS	1.5 T Siemens	cs-fMRI	NA	DBS ON/OFF	SI, SII, Th, In, CC

Jones et al. (2021) [53]	PS-pain (5); HC (6)	VS/ ALIC	8 months 11 months	3 T Siemens	tb-fMRI	Heat stimuli	DBS ON/OFF x stimuli x (Un)/Affected side x DBS/HC	Th, In, Op, OFC, SCC, Hc
Middlebrooks et al. (2020) [54]	Epilepsy (2)	ANT	1–3 months	1.5 T Siemens	cs-fMRI	NA	DBS ON/OFF	Th, ACC, PCC, PCn, mPFC, Am, VTA, Hc, St, AG
Middlebrooks et al. (2021) [55]	Epilepsy (5)	ANT	2–8 months	1.5 T Siemens	cs-fMRI	NA	DBS ON/OFF x Stimulation frequency	Hc, ACC, Am, ANT, mPFC, VTA, PCC, PCn, AG, PHG, mThal, BFor, NAc
Sarica et al. (2021) [56]	Epilepsy (2)	ANT	1 day (1), 4 years (1)	3 T GE	cs-fMRI	NA	DBS ON/OFF	Th, VTA
Jo et al. (2018) [57]	TS (5)	CMPf	Intra-op; 1 week	1.5 T GE	cs-fMRI	NA	NA	FSN, LN, MN, FN, PN
Gratwicke et al. (2020) [58]	LBD (6)	NBM	6 weeks, 20 weeks	1.5 T Siemens	rs-fMRI	NA	DBS ON/OFF	CC, iPL, DMN, FPN, IPS, IPG, PCn, PCG

[a]Rezai et al. (1999) was reported twice in this table as a study that included essential tremor and refractory pain patients. Modified from [59]

ACC anterior cingulate cortex, *AG* angular gyrus, *ALIC* anterior limb of the internal capsule, *Am* amygdala, *ANT* anterior nucleus of the thalamus, *BGe* basal ganglia externa, *BS* brainstem, *BFor* basal forebrain, *Ca* caudate, *CC* cingulate cortex, *Cer* cerebellum, *CMPf* thalamic centromedian parafascicular complex, *CN* caudate nucleus, *CSC* cortico-striatal connectivity, *CSTC* cortico-subthalamic nucleus connectivity, *CTCC* cortico-thalamo-cerebellar network, *cs* cycling-stimulation, *cZI* caudal zona incerta, *d* days, *dACC* dorsal anterior cingulate, *DBS* deep brain stimulation, *LBD* Lewy body dementia, *DLPFC* dorsolateral prefrontal cortex, *DMN* default mode network, *ET* essential tremor, *fMRI* functional magnetic resonance imaging, *FN* frontal network, *FPN* frontoparietal network, *Fr* frontal lobule, *FSN* frontostriatal network, *GE* General Electric, *GPe* globus pallidus externus, *GPi* globus pallidus internus, *HC* healthy controls,

(continued)

Table 7.1 (continued)

Hc hippocampus, *i* inferior, *IFG* inferior frontal gyrus, *In* insular cortex, *IPL* inferior parietal lobule, *IPS* intraparietal sulcus, *LFS* low-frequency stimulation, *LN* limbic network, *LPMC* lateral premotor cortex, *m* medial, *M1* primary visual cortex, *MC* motor cortex, *MN* motor network, *NA* not applicable, *NAc* nucleus accumbens, *NS* not specified, *Occ* occipital lobe, *OCD* obsessive-compulsive disorder, *OFC* orbitofrontal cortex, *op* operative, *Op* operculum, *PCC* posterior cingulate cortex, *PCG* paracingulate gyrus, *PCG* precentral gyrus, *PCn* precuneus, *PD* Parkinson's disease, *PF* prefrontal cortex, *PL* parietal lobule, *PM* primary motor, *PMC* premotor cortex, *PN* parietal network, *Po* pons, *PPN* pedunculopontine nucleus, *PS* post-stroke, *Pu* putamen, *PVG* periventricular gray, *RF* radiofrequency, *rs* resting state, *SC* superior colliculus, *SCC* superior convexity cortex, *SI* primary somatosensory cortex, *SII* secondary somatosensory cortex, *SMA* supplementary motor area, *SMC* sensorimotor cortex, *SMCC* sensorimotor cortex-cerebellar connectivity, *SMG* supramarginal gyrus, *SN* substantia nigra, *SSC* striatal-subthalamic nucleus connectivity, *st* stimulation task, *St* striatum, *STC* striato-thalamic connectivity, *SNTC* subthalamic nucleus-thalamic connectivity, *STN* subthalamic nucleus, *T* tesla, *Th* thalamus, *TS* Tourette syndrome, *VC* ventral capsule, *VIM* ventral intermediate nucleus, VS ventral striatal, VS ventral striatum, *VTA* ventral tegmental area, *w/* with, *WMT* white matter tracts

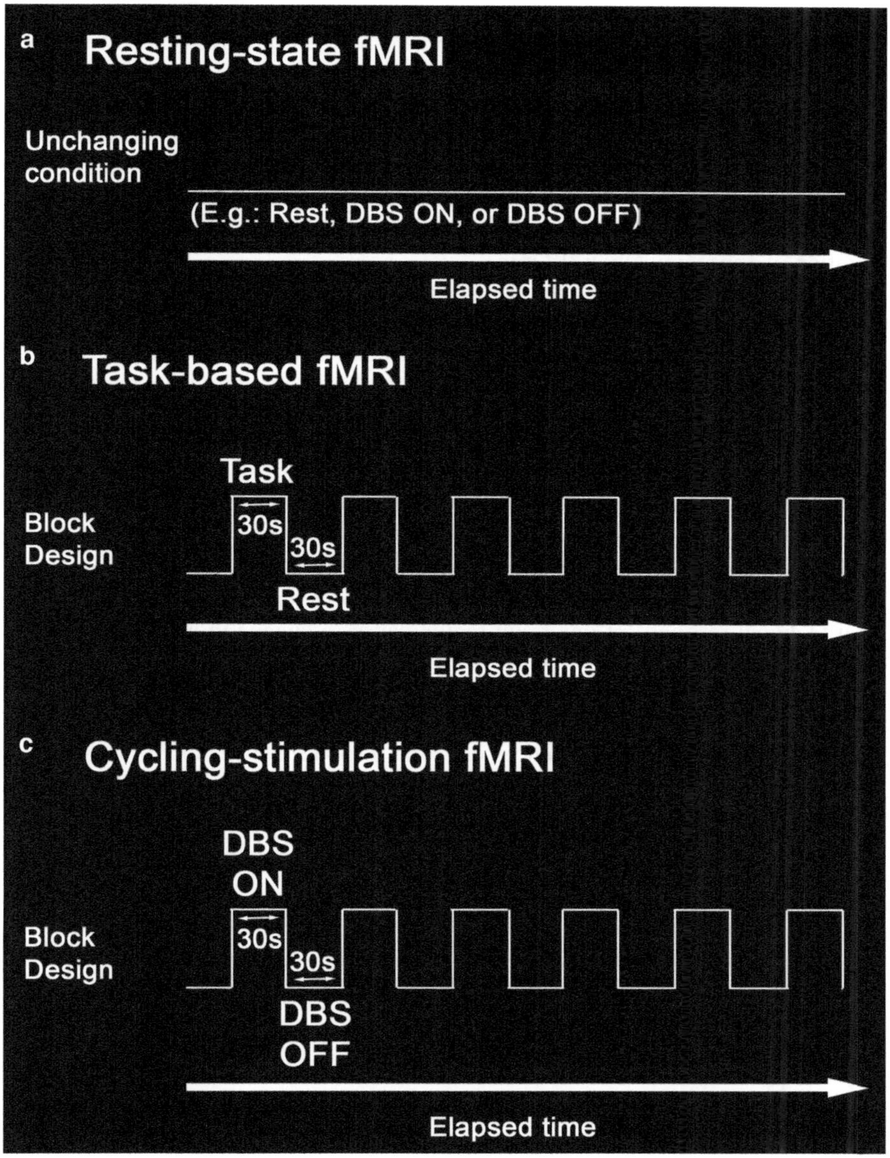

Fig. 7.3 Schematic representation of fMRI-DBS experimental design and acquisition. (**a**) Resting-state fMRI involves acquiring scans when subjects at rest and the experimental or stimulation conditions remain constant throughout the duration of the scan. (**b**) Task-based fMRI involves acquiring scans while participants perform tasks specifically designed to induce cognitive changes. "Block design" is a specific paradigm in which participants alternate between a period of performing a task, followed by a period of rest in a continuous ON/OFF fashion. (**c**) Cycling-stimulation fMRI is an extension of task-based block-design fMRI, where DBS is programmed to cycle between different conditions in a continuous ON/OFF fashion

studies included in this review that employed the task-based fMRI paradigm used the block design, where participants alternate between a period of performing a task, followed by a period of rest (control), continuously. Finally, cycling-stimulation fMRI is an extension of block-design fMRI. It involves programming the stimulation to cycle between different conditions (e.g., DBS ON and OFF or optimal and non-optimal settings). Comparable with task-based fMRI studies, studies that employ the cycling-stimulation fMRI paradigm programmed the DBS device to alternate between DBS ON and OFF states for 15–30 second intervals, for a total duration of approximately 6–12 min.

Researchers can employ one of many statistical tools to analyze their data. The specific analytical approach used by each study will differ based on the study's research question and hypothesis, as well as their fMRI experimental design and acquisition. In total, ten fMRI-DBS studies employed a resting-state experimental design. These studies predominantly investigate functional connectivity, which show undirected temporal associations between the BOLD signal from distinct brain regions or across the whole brain [27, 37, 43, 47, 52, 58, 60]. There were many methods to analyze resting-state networks including seed or region-of-interest based analysis, correlation analysis, whole-brain computational modeling, and eigenvector centrality modeling [9, 10]. rs-fMRI DBS studies have also employed dynamic causal modeling to investigate effective connectivity, that is how the BOLD signal response of one brain region causes a change in another, as well as amplitude of low-frequency fluctuations (ALFF) which reflects the regional intensity of spontaneous fluctuations in the BOLD signal [24, 35, 36, 52].

Eleven fMRI-DBS studies employed task-based fMRI paradigms. These studies commonly examined the differences in neural response between two states or conditions (e.g., task vs rest) using Student's T-tests, general linear modeling, regression analysis, or a combination of these methods [28–31, 41, 50, 53]. These methods can be used to create contrast or "activation" maps that show brain regions with BOLD signal changes that are significantly associated with the two conditions [9, 10]. A small number of task-based fMRI-DBS studies examined connectivity [32, 35, 36, 48]. Since the cycling-stimulation fMRI paradigm (n = 21) is an extension of task-based fMRI, cycling-stimulation fMRI-DBS studies employed similar fMRI analysis techniques used in task-based fMRI studies to identify changes in BOLD signals significantly associated with DBS.

Movement Disorders

Parkinson's Disease (PD)

PD is the most common DBS indication investigated by fMRI. For the treatment of PD, DBS electrodes are placed in major hubs of the motor circuit such as the subthalami nucleus (STN) and the globus pallidus pars interna (GPi). Two-thirds (n = 24) of studies reviewed in this chapter included PD patients treated

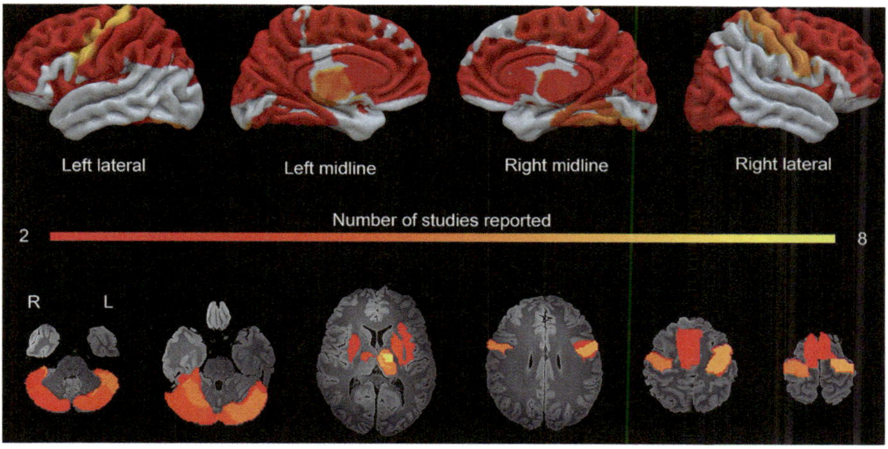

Fig. 7.4 BOLD signal changes associated with STN-DBS acquired using cycling-stimulation fMRI. Results only from cycling-stimulation fMRI-DBS were included in this figure because these studies intuitively report brain regions where STN stimulation increased or decreased BOLD signal, whereas task-based fMRI report BOLD signal effects due to DBS and motor tasks and resting-state fMRI report changes in connectivity. Studies reporting brain areas modulated by STN-DBS using a cycling-stimulation fMRI paradigm were identified. These areas were assigned an automated anatomical labeling 3 (AAL3) atlas parcellation based on their reported MNI or Talairach coordinates, or their qualitative description. Across all studies, the frequency that each AAL3 (https://bioimagesuiteweb.github.io/webapp/mni2tal.html) region was reported was used as a weighting (e.g. if the right Pallidum – AAL3 region 80 – was reported in 5 studies, it was assigned a value of 5). Weighted parcellations were then used to generate a frequency map, which was overlaid on axial slices of a standard MNI T1-weighted brain template (https://www.bic.mni.mcgill.ca/ServicesAtlases/ICBM152NLin2009). Only brain regions that were reported by three or more publications were included in the figure. The color gradient represents the number of studies. The most-reported areas (yellow) include thalamus ($n = 8$), M1 ($n = 6$), and palladium ($n = 6$). Sum map was overlayed on BrainMesh_ICBM 152 brain available on the software Surf Ice v1 (https://github.com/neurolabusc/surf-ice), and overlayed on a standard MNI T1-weighted brain template (https://www.nature.com/articles/s41597-019-0254-8) and visualized using FSLeyes

STN-DBS. Three of these studies included a smaller cohort of PD patients treated with GPi-DBS.

The most common experimental design used in PD fMRI-DBS studies was the cycling-stimulation paradigm ($n = 10$ studies). These studies identified brain regions associated with DBS ON and OFF conditions [22, 25, 26, 33, 39, 40, 42, 44–46]. Cycling between DBS ON and OFF states was associated with BOLD signal changes in the motor cortex, cerebellum, and the basal ganglia, including the thalamus, globus pallidus (GP), substantia nigra, and caudate nucleus (Fig. 7.4). In particular, the BOLD signal of the GP and thalamus consistently increased in the STN-DBS ON state when compared to OFF [22, 25, 26, 39, 40, 44–46]. However, the directions of BOLD signal changes of other brain regions were variable. For example, the BOLD signal of the premotor cortex and M1 was reported to increase with STN stimulation [33, 39, 40, 42, 46], but three papers with large sample sizes reported decreased BOLD response from M1 [22, 26, 45]. Likewise, the cerebellum showed both increased [25, 26, 40, 42, 44–46] and decreased [22, 26, 44, 45] BOLD response to STN stimulation.

Though the reasons for these discrepancies are unclear, differences in BOLD signal response to STN-DBS may be attributable to differences in scanning conditions (e.g., awake vs general anesthesia; medication status at the time of scan), stimulation parameters (e.g., optimal vs suboptimal stimulation), variability in the biological response to stimulation across individuals, and specific patient characteristics (e.g., PD phenotype). Knight et al. [42] reported that DBS induced similar brain regions in both the awake and anesthesia state; however, BOLD signal intensity was stronger when subjects were awake. Variations in BOLD signal response may also be attributable to DBS stimulation settings. Indeed, frequency-dependent BOLD signal responses have been reported in GP, thalamus, and cerebellum [44, 45]. Boutet et al. [22] reported that clinically suboptimal stimulation parameters (i.e. voltage, frequency, and contact) produce a different BOLD fMRI signal signature than that produced by clinically optimal settings. Additionally, Hancu et al. [26] reported subject-level differences in BOLD signal response between monopolar and bipolar STN stimulation. Another possible explanation for BOLD signal variability in cycling-stimulation fMRI studies is PD phenotype. Dimarzio et al. [33] reported that STN-DBS induced increased M1 BOLD response among patients with akinesia-rigidity type PD and decreased response in patients with tremor dominant PD.

In addition to cycling-stimulation fMRI-DBS studies, eight studies employed rs-fMRI in PD patients to investigate the impact of STN-DBS on neural networks and functional connectivity [24, 27, 32, 34, 35, 37, 61]. STN stimulation was consistently shown to modulate brain areas associated with the cortico-striato-thalamic-cortical loop. STN-DBS was commonly associated with increased connections within and between M1, supplementary motor area, striatum, thalamus, cerebellum, and putamen [24, 32, 34, 35, 47, 61]. STN-DBS was also found to reduce the strength of all STN afferent and efferent projections and connections between the STN and thalamus [35, 36]. Interestingly, two studies with age-matched healthy controls showed that STN-DBS normalized the global brain connectivity patterns of PD patients to that of healthy controls, suggesting that the therapeutic mechanism of DBS involves modulations of large-scale brain networks as well as changes to local brain activation [27, 37].

Eight studies employed task-based fMRI to investigate BOLD signal changes associated with DBS during motor or sensory tasks. Hesselmen et al. [41] showed that STN-DBS during finger-tapping task increased BOLD signal in the anterior insula, putamen, and caudate nucleus and decreased signal in the primary sensory motor cortex and cerebellum when compared with DBS OFF. Furthermore, effective connectivity studies reported that STN-DBS modulated the cortico-striato-thalamic-cortical loop and recruited subcortical-cerebellar pathways during voluntary movement tasks [35, 36]. In contrast, Mueller et al. [30] found no significant interactions between STN-DBS and motor tasks. Of note, Steinhardt et al. [48] found that the STN-DBS increased the functional connectivity of the salience network and simultaneously decreased the connectivity of reward-related networks in the context of food cue processing.

Among these studies, three included smaller cohorts of PD patients treated with GPi-DBS [22, 33, 47]. A cycling-stimulation fMRI study by Dimarzio et al. [33] found that both STN and GPi stimulation increased the BOLD signal in the thalamus and GP. Conversely, GPi stimulation was associated with decreased BOLD signal of the M1, whereas STN stimulation increased M1 signal. A recent rs-fMRI study showed that both STN and GPi-DBS reduced the functional connectivity among motor-related cortical and subcortical regions. However, STN-DBS showed a more extensive reduction in connectivity between the postcentral gyrus and the cerebellar vermis [47].

Essential Tremor (ET)

Besides PD, BOLD fMRI has been used to investigate the effects of DBS in ET [23, 29, 38]. The first of the studies acquired fMRI from two ET patients with ventral intermediate thalamus (VIM) DBS while stimulation cycled between ON and OFF states. VIM stimulation induced BOLD signal responses in the thalamus, basal ganglia, and somatosensory cortex [23]. Seventeen years later, another study acquired intraoperative fMRI from 10 ET patients with VIM-DBS using a cycling-stimulation fMRI paradigm. The authors observed that VIM-DBS was associated with significant BOLD response in the sensorimotor cortex, thalamus, and cerebellum and that their BOLD response was positively correlated with therapeutic effect [38]. Most recently, Awad et al. [29] acquired fMRI from 16 patients with caudal zona incerta (cZI) DBS while participants engaged in motor tasks using a task-based fMRI paradigm. Independent of motor tasks, cZI-DBS modulated the BOLD response of the premotor cortex, while task-dependent DBS effects were observed in the primary sensorimotor cortex (S1), supplementary motor area, and cerebellum [29].

Neuropsychiatric Disorders

Obsessive-Compulsive Disorder (OCD)

As of yet, very few publications have used fMRI to investigate the effect of DBS on BOLD signal changes and connectivity outside of movement disorders. Three studies have assessed the effect of DBS using fMRI in OCD [49–51]. A case report of an OCD patient treated with bilateral nucleus accumbens (NAc) DBS found local BOLD signal changes in the medial thalamus, putamen, head of the caudate, anterior cingulate, and the cerebellum using cycling-stimulation fMRI [49]. In a subsequent case series, three OCD patients received NAc-DBS and an intraoperative fMRI using the cycling-stimulation fMRI paradigm [50]. The study investigated BOLD response to both NAc and internal capsule stimulation by changing the stimulation location using different contacts. Stimulation of the internal capsule was associated with subject-level BOLD signal changes in the caudate nucleus and anterior cingulum. NAc stimulation was associated with

BOLD signal changes in the limbic system, including the parahippocampal region which was common to all three patients [50]. Gibson et al. [51] examined the BOLD signal response to laughter-inducing ventral capsule/ventral striatum (VC/VS) stimulation in four OCD patients under general anesthesia using rs-fMRI. Stimulation of the VC/VS was associated with BOLD signal changes in the mediodorsal thalamus, amygdala, pons, and orbitofrontal cortex. Interestingly, laughter-inducing stimulation was associated with enhanced connectivity from the anterior cingulate cortex to VS and attenuated connectivity from the thalamus to VS.

Depression, Anorexia, and Bipolar

More recently, Elias et al. [52] employed resting-state fMRI to investigate subcallosal cingulate (SCC) DBS within 16 patients with major depressive disorder, anorexia nervosa, or bipolar. ALFF analysis found that SCC-DBS reduced spontaneous changes in BOLD signal in the bilateral dorsal anterior cingulate cortex, posterior cingulate cortex, precuneus, middle cingulate cortex, middle frontal gyrus, left inferior parietal lobule, and lateral occipital cortex. Interestingly, the study found that ALFF BOLD signal changes in the dorsal ACC, left PCC, and left precuneus significantly predicted clinical improvement. Additionally, functional connectivity analysis found that SCC-DBS increased the connectedness between the above regions.

Pain

The effect of DBS on pain has been investigated by three studies [23, 28, 53]. Two of the studies scanned participants while stimulation was cycling between DBS ON vs OFF states. The first included three subjects with refractory chronic pain treated with ventralis caudalis nucleus of the thalamus (Vc) (n = 2) and periventricular gray (PVG) DBS (n = 1). While Vc stimulation increased the BOLD signal of the somatosensory perception pathways including the S1 and secondary somatosensory cortex (S2), thalamus, and insula, PVG stimulation only increased the BOLD signal in the anterior cingulate cortex and the medial thalamus [23]. A subsequent paper examined BOLD signal changes associated with STN stimulation in PD patients with chronic pain. The study reported that STN stimulation was associated with increased BOLD signal in the S1 cortex among participants experiencing pain relief (n = 5) and decreased S1 BOLD signal in treatment non-responders (n = 5), suggesting that differential BOLD response of S1 may be a potential fMRI signature for pain relief [28].

Jones et al. [53] applied heat stimuli to 10 patients with post-stroke pain syndrome treated with the anterior limb of the internal capsule (ALIC) DBS. Heat stimuli were delivered to patients in a block paradigm during both DBS ON and OFF conditions. In the DBS OFF state, heat stimuli were associated with increased BOLD response of the orbitofrontal and superior convexity cortex. When

ALIC-DBS was turned ON, the signal from these regions was reduced and fewer foci were reported in response to heat stimuli. Additionally, heat stimuli were associated with decreased BOLD response of the precentral gyrus and hippocampus with ALIC stimulation.

Epilepsy

Three fMRI studies have evaluated the effects of anterior thalamic nucleus (ANT) stimulation for the treatment of epilepsy [54–56]. Cycling-stimulation fMRI in four patients treated with ANT stimulation showed a widespread increase in BOLD signal within the default mode network (DMN) and limbic network including the thalamus, anterior and posterior cingulate cortex, precuneus, medial prefrontal cortex, amygdala, ventral tegmental area, hippocampus, striatum, and right angular gyrus [54]. Changing the active stimulation contact away from ANT reduced the BOLD signal intensity of these areas [56] and high-frequency (145 Hz) ANT-DBS produced greater BOLD signal increase within the DMN and limbic networks compared to low-frequency stimulation (30 Hz) [55].

Other DBS Indications

Other DBS indications investigated using fMRI included Lewy body dementia (LBD) [58] and TS [57]. In a randomized, crossover, double-blind trial, four LBD participants with DBS of the nucleus basalis of Meynert (NBM) underwent resting-state fMRI. In these patients, NBM stimulation was associated with decreased connectivity within the DMN, specifically between the posterior cingulate cortex and the right inferior parietal lobule. NBM stimulation was also associated with changes in the functional connectivity of the frontoparietal network. Finally, Jo et al. [57] examined the effects of stimulating the centromedian nucleus of the thalamus in five TS patients using cycling-stimulation fMRI. The authors reported that thalamic DBS induced suppression of the motor and insular networks which was associated with motor tic reduction. Likewise, stimulation suppressed frontal and parietal networks which was associated with vocal tic reduction.

Potential Applications and Future Directions

The fMRI-DBS literature is a rapidly growing field in the world of functional neuroimaging. Half the number of papers reviewed by this book chapter were published in the last five years and the number of fMRI-DBS studies published each year is steadily increasing. While these fMRI-DBS studies have traditionally focused on elucidating neural responses to stimulation, more recent studies have assessed the potential of fMRI as a clinical tool to improve DBS treatment. Among PD DBS patients, fMRI has been used to identify specific BOLD activation and connectivity signatures associated with optimal and suboptimal DBS parameters. These signatures could be used to better direct DBS programming, which is currently a time-intensive process based on subjective evaluations of patient-specific responses to stimulation. Additionally, future DBS-fMRI studies could use intraoperative fMRI to assess real-time modulation of brain activity and recruitment of neural networks during DBS implantation. Thus, intraoperative fMRI could supplement electrophysiological local field potential recordings to better guide DBS targeting.

Furthermore, there are many DBS indications and targets that have yet to be investigated by fMRI. Outside of PD, limited studies have been published for each DBS indication, often with small sample sizes. DBS indications that have yet to be explored by fMRI include dystonia, Alzheimer's disease, and consciousness disorders. fMRI may offer valuable insights within these conditions, further supplementing findings from other functional imaging modalities. Combining DBS with fMRI provides a unique opportunity to probe and modulate neural circuits and interrogate dynamic neural responses to stimulation. As DBS hardware and fMRI technology and analysis continue to advance, fMRI-DBS studies may offer opportunities to not just understand the mechanisms of DBS, but to better understand neuropsychiatric diseases and ultimately the complexities of the brain.

References

1. Chiken S, Nambu A. Mechanism of deep brain stimulation: inhibition, excitation, or disruption? Neuroscientist. 2016;22(3):313–22.
2. Lozano AM, Lipsman N. Probing and regulating dysfunctional circuits using deep brain stimulation. Neuron. 2013;77(3):406–24.
3. Fenoy AJ, Simpson RK Jr. Risks of common complications in deep brain stimulation surgery: management and avoidance. J Neurosurg. 2014;120(1):132–9.
4. Lozano AM, Lipsman N, Bergman H, Brown P, Chabardes S, Chang JW, et al. Deep brain stimulation: current challenges and future directions. Nat Rev Neurol. 2019;15(3):148–60.
5. Litvak V, Florin E, Tamás G, Groppa S, Muthuraman M. EEG and MEG primers for tracking DBS network effects. NeuroImage. 2021;224:117447.
6. Sui Y, Tian Y, Ko WKD, Wang Z, Jia F, Horn A, et al. Deep brain stimulation initiative: toward innovative technology, new disease indications, and approaches to current and future clinical challenges in neuromodulation therapy. Front Neurol. 2020;11:597451.
7. Boutet A, Jain M, Gwun D, Rusjan P, Neudorfer C, Elias GJB, et al. Modulation of CNS functions by deep brain stimulation: insights provided by molecular imaging. In: Dierckx RAJO, Otte A, de Vries EFJ, van Waarde A, Leenders KL, editors. PET and SPECT in neurology. Cham: Springer International Publishing; 2021. p. 1177–244.
8. Ko JH, Tang CC, Eidelberg D. Brain stimulation and functional imaging with fMRI and PET. Handb Clin Neurol. 2013;116:77–95.
9. Glover GH. Overview of functional magnetic resonance imaging. Neurosurg Clin N Am. 2011;22(2):133–9. vii
10. Soares JM, Magalhães R, Moreira PS, Sousa A, Ganz E, Sampaio A, et al. A Hitchhiker's guide to functional magnetic resonance imaging [internet]. Vol. 10, Front Neurosci. 2016. https://doi.org/10.3389/fnins.2016.00515.
11. Boutet A, Chow CT, Narang K, Elias GJB, Neudorfer C, Germann J, et al. Improving safety of MRI in patients with deep brain stimulation devices. Radiology. 2020;296(2):250–62.
12. Boutet A, Hancu I, Saha U, Crawley A, Xu DS, Ranjan M, et al. 3-tesla MRI of deep brain stimulation patients: safety assessment of coils and pulse sequences. J Neurosurg. 2019;132(2):586–94.

13. Boutet A, Rashid T, Hancu I, Elias GJB, Gramer RM, Germann J, et al. Functional MRI safety and artifacts during deep brain stimulation: experience in 102 patients. Radiology. 2019;293(1):174–83.
14. Horn A, Blankenburg F. Toward a standardized structural-functional group connectome in MNI space. NeuroImage. 2016;124(Pt A):310–22.
15. Horn A, Kühn AA, Merkl A, Shih L, Alterman R, Fox M. Probabilistic conversion of neurosurgical DBS electrode coordinates into MNI space. NeuroImage. 2017;150:395–404.
16. Wang Q, Akram H, Muthuraman M, Gonzalez-Escamilla G, Sheth SA, Oxenford S, et al. Normative vs. patient-specific brain connectivity in deep brain stimulation. NeuroImage. 2021;224:117307.
17. Wong JK, Middlebrooks EH, Grewal SS, Almeida L, Hess CW, Okun MS. A comprehensive review of brain Connectomics and imaging to improve deep brain stimulation outcomes. Mov Disord. 2020;35(5):741–51.
18. Elias GJB, Germann J, Loh A, Boutet A, Taha A, Wong EHY, et al. Chapter 12—normative connectomes and their use in DBS. In: Horn A, editor. Connectomic deep brain stimulation. Academic Press; 2022. p. 245–74.
19. Germann J, Zadeh G, Mansouri A, Kucharczyk W, Lozano AM, Boutet A. Untapped neuroimaging tools for neuro-oncology: connectomics and spatial transcriptomics. Cancers [Internet]. 2022;14:3. https://doi.org/10.3390/cancers14030464.
20. Horn A, Reich M, Vorwerk J, Li N, Wenzel G, Fang Q, et al. Connectivity predicts deep brain stimulation outcome in Parkinson disease. Ann Neurol. 2017;82(1):67–78.
21. Fox MD. Mapping symptoms to brain networks with the human connectome. N Engl J Med. 2018;379(23):2237–45.
22. Boutet A, Madhavan R, Elias GJB, Joel SE, Gramer R, Ranjan M, et al. Predicting optimal deep brain stimulation parameters for Parkinson's disease using functional MRI and machine learning. Nat Commun. 2021;12(1):3043.
23. Rezai AR, Lozano AM, Crawley AP, Joy ML, Davis KD, Kwan CL, et al. Thalamic stimulation and functional magnetic resonance imaging: localization of cortical and subcortical activation with implanted electrodes. Technical note. J Neurosurg. 1999;90(3):583–90.
24. Hanssen H, Steinhardt J, Münchau A, Al-Zubaidi A, Tzvi E, Heldmann M, et al. Cerebello-striatal interaction mediates effects of subthalamic nucleus deep brain stimulation in Parkinson's disease. Parkinsonism Relat Disord. 2019;67:99–104.
25. Phillips MD, Baker KB, Lowe MJ, Tkach JA, Cooper SE, Kopell BH, et al. Parkinson disease: pattern of functional MR imaging activation during deep brain stimulation of subthalamic nucleus—initial experience. Radiology. 2006;239(1):209–16.
26. Hancu I, Boutet A, Fiveland E, Ranjan M, Prusik J, Dimarzio M, et al. On the (non-)equivalency of monopolar and bipolar settings for deep brain stimulation fMRI studies of Parkinson's disease patients. J Magn Reson Imaging. 2019;49(6):1736–49.
27. Saenger VM, Kahan J, Foltynie T, Friston K, Aziz TZ, Green AL, et al. Uncovering the underlying mechanisms and whole-brain dynamics of deep brain stimulation for Parkinson's disease. Sci Rep. 2017;7(1):9882.
28. DiMarzio M, Rashid T, Hancu I, Fiveland E, Prusik J, Gillogly M, et al. Functional MRI signature of chronic pain relief from deep brain stimulation in Parkinson disease patients. Neurosurgery. 2019;85(6):E1043–9.
29. Awad A, Blomstedt P, Westling G, Eriksson J. Deep brain stimulation in the caudal zona incerta modulates the sensorimotor cerebello-cerebral circuit in essential tremor. NeuroImage. 2020;209:116511.
30. Mueller K, Urgošík D, Ballarini T, Holiga Š, Möller HE, Růžička F, et al. Differential effects of deep brain stimulation and levodopa on brain activity in Parkinson's disease. Brain Commun. 2020;2(1):fcaa005.
31. Arantes PR, Cardoso EF, Barreiros MA, Teixeira MJ, Gonçalves MR, Barbosa ER, et al. Performing functional magnetic resonance imaging in patients with Parkinson's disease treated with deep brain stimulation. Mov Disord. 2006;21(8):1154–62.

32. Kahan J, Mancini L, Urner M, Friston K, Hariz M, Holl E, et al. Therapeutic subthalamic nucleus deep brain stimulation reverses cortico-thalamic coupling during voluntary movements in Parkinson's disease. PLoS One. 2012;7(12):e50270.
33. DiMarzio M, Madhavan R, Joel S, Hancu I, Fiveland E, Prusik J, et al. Use of functional magnetic resonance imaging to assess how motor phenotypes of Parkinson's disease respond to deep brain stimulation [internet]. Neuromodulation: Technology at the Neural Interface. 2020;23:515–24. https://doi.org/10.1111/ner.13160.
34. Holiga Š, Mueller K, Möller HE, Urgošík D, Růžička E, Schroeter ML, et al. Resting-state functional magnetic resonance imaging of the subthalamic microlesion and stimulation effects in Parkinson's disease: indications of a principal role of the brainstem. Neuroimage Clin. 2015;9:264–74.
35. Kahan J, Urner M, Moran R, Flandin G, Marreiros A, Mancini L, et al. Resting state functional MRI in Parkinson's disease: the impact of deep brain stimulation on "effective" connectivity. Brain. 2014;137(4):1130–44.
36. Kahan J, Mancini L, Flandin G, White M, Papadaki A, Thornton J, et al. Deep brain stimulation has state-dependent effects on motor connectivity in Parkinson's disease [internet]. Brain. 2019;142:2417–31. https://doi.org/10.1093/brain/awz164.
37. Horn A, Wenzel G, Irmen F, Huebl J, Li N, Neumann W-J, et al. Deep brain stimulation induced normalization of the human functional connectome in Parkinson's disease. Brain. 2019;142(10):3129–43.
38. Gibson WS, Jo HJ, Testini P, Cho S, Felmlee JP, Welker KM, et al. Functional correlates of the therapeutic and adverse effects evoked by thalamic stimulation for essential tremor. Brain. 2016;139(Pt 8):2198–210.
39. Jech R, Urgosík D, Tintera J, Nebuzelský A, Krásenský J, Liscák R, et al. Functional magnetic resonance imaging during deep brain stimulation: a pilot study in four patients with Parkinson's disease. Mov Disord. 2001;16(6):1126–32.
40. Stefurak T, Mikulis D, Mayberg H, Lang AE, Hevenor S, Pahapill P, et al. Deep brain stimulation for Parkinson's disease dissociates mood and motor circuits: a functional MRI case study. Mov Disord. 2003;18(12):1508–16.
41. Hesselmann V, Sorger B, Girnus R, Lasek K, Maarouf M, Wedekind C, et al. Intraoperative functional MRI as a new approach to monitor deep brain stimulation in Parkinson's disease. Eur Radiol. 2004;14(4):686–90.
42. Knight EJ, Testini P, Min H-K, Gibson WS, Gorny KR, Favazza CP, et al. Motor and nonmotor circuitry activation induced by subthalamic nucleus deep brain stimulation in patients with Parkinson disease: intraoperative functional magnetic resonance imaging for deep brain stimulation. Mayo Clin Proc. 2015;90(6):773–85.
43. Mueller K, Jech R, Růžička F, Holiga Š, Ballarini T, Bezdicek O, et al. Brain connectivity changes when comparing effects of subthalamic deep brain stimulation with levodopa treatment in Parkinson's disease. Neuroimage Clin. 2018;19:1025–35.
44. DiMarzio M, Madhavan R, Hancu I, Fiveland E, Prusik J, Joel S, et al. Use of functional MRI to assess effects of deep brain stimulation frequency changes on brain activation in Parkinson disease. Neurosurgery. 2021;88(2):356–65.
45. Shen L, Jiang C, Hubbard CS, Ren J, He C, Wang D, et al. Subthalamic nucleus deep brain stimulation modulates 2 distinct neurocircuits. Ann Neurol. 2020;88(6):1178–93.
46. Gibson WS, Rusheen AE, Oh Y, In M-H, Gorny KR, Felmlee JP, et al. Symptom-specific differential motor network modulation by deep brain stimulation in Parkinson's disease. J Neurosurg. 2021:1–9.
47. Zhang C, Lai Y, Li J, He N, Liu Y, Li Y, et al. Subthalamic and pallidal stimulations in patients with Parkinson's disease: common and dissociable connections. Ann Neurol. 2021;90(4):670–82.
48. Steinhardt J, Hanssen H, Heldmann M, Neumann A, Münchau A, Schramm P, et al. Sweets for my sweet: modulation of the limbic system drives salience for sweet foods after deep brain stimulation in Parkinson's disease. J Neurol Neurosurg Psychiatry [Internet]. 2021; https://doi.org/10.1136/jnnp-2021-326280.

49. Baker KB, Kopell BH, Malone D, Horenstein C, Lowe M, Phillips MD, et al. Deep brain stimulation for obsessive-compulsive disorder: using functional magnetic resonance imaging and electrophysiological techniques: technical case report. Neurosurgery. 2007;61(5 Suppl 2):E367–8. discussion E368.
50. Hiss S, Hesselmann V, Hunsche S, Kugel H, Sturm V, Maintz D, et al. Intraoperative functional magnetic resonance imaging for monitoring the effect of deep brain stimulation in patients with obsessive-compulsive disorder. Stereotact Funct Neurosurg. 2015;93(1):30–7.
51. Gibson WS, Cho S, Abulseoud OA, Gorny KR, Felmlee JP, Welker KM, et al. The impact of mirth-inducing ventral striatal deep brain stimulation on functional and effective connectivity. Cereb Cortex. 2017;27(3):2183–94.
52. Elias GJB, Germann J, Boutet A, Loh A, Li B, Pancholi A, et al. 3 T MRI of rapid brain activity changes driven by subcallosal cingulate deep brain stimulation. Brain [Internet]. 2021; https://doi.org/10.1093/brain/awab447.
53. Jones SE, Lempka SF, Gopalakrishnan R, Baker KB, Beall EB, Bhattacharyya P, et al. Functional magnetic resonance imaging correlates of ventral striatal deep brain stimulation for poststroke pain. Neuromodulation. 2021;24(2):259–64.
54. Middlebrooks EH, Lin C, Okromelidze L, Lu C-Q, Tatum WO, Wharen RE Jr, et al. Functional activation patterns of deep brain stimulation of the anterior nucleus of the thalamus. World Neurosurg. 2020;136:357–63.e2.
55. Middlebrooks EH, Jain A, Okromelidze L, Lin C, Westerhold EM, O'Steen CA, et al. Acute brain activation patterns of high- versus low-frequency stimulation of the anterior nucleus of the thalamus during deep brain stimulation for epilepsy. Neurosurgery. 2021;89(5):901–8.
56. Sarica C, Yamamoto K, Loh A, Elias GJB, Boutet A, Madhavan R, et al. Blood oxygen level-dependent (BOLD) response patterns with thalamic deep brain stimulation in patients with medically refractory epilepsy. Epilepsy Behav. 2021;122:108153.
57. Jo HJ, McCairn KW, Gibson WS, Testini P, Zhao CZ, Gorny KR, et al. Global network modulation during thalamic stimulation for Tourette syndrome. Neuroimage Clin. 2018;18:502–9.
58. Gratwicke J, Zrinzo L, Kahan J, Peters A, Brechany U, McNichol A, et al. Bilateral nucleus basalis of Meynert deep brain stimulation for dementia with Lewy bodies: a randomised clinical trial. Brain Stimul. 2020;13(4):1031–9.
59. Loh A, Gwun D, Chow CT, Boutet A, Tasserie J, Germann J, et al. Probing responses to deep brain stimulation with functional magnetic resonance imaging. Brain Stimul. 2022;5(3):683–94.
60. Holiga Š, Mueller K, Möller HE, Urgošík D, Růžička E, Schroeter ML, et al. Resting-state functional magnetic resonance imaging of the subthalamic microlesion and stimulation effects in Parkinson's disease: indications of a principal role of the brainstem [internet]. NeuroImage Clin. 2015;9:264–74. https://doi.org/10.1016/j.nicl.2015.08.008.
61. Kahan J, Mancini L, Flandin G, White M, Papadaki A, Thornton J, et al. Deep brain stimulation has state-dependent effects on motor connectivity in Parkinson's disease. Brain. 2019;142(8):2417–31.

MRI in Pediatric Patients Undergoing DBS

8

Han Yan, Elysa Widjaja, Carolina Gorodetsky, and George M. Ibrahim

Introduction

As with most novel technologies and innovations within medicine, deep brain stimulation (DBS) became a commonplace tool first for adults prior to being applied to pediatric patients. One of the earliest reports of DBS for a child took place in November, 1996 [1]. Bilateral stimulation of the globus pallidus interna (GPi) was offered to an 8-year-old girl with severe generalized dystonia, who had been under sedation and respiratory assistance for 2 months prior to the surgery. DBS helped her recovery with lasting benefits for 20 years [2].

The indications for pediatric DBS slowly began to expand despite the challenges related to the lack of pediatric-specific clinical trials. Nonetheless, there are special considerations concerning DBS surgery for children and adolescents; and there are also unique considerations regarding the acquisition, use, and study of magnetic resonance imaging (MRI) for these patients.

This chapter will introduce the specific indications of DBS for children and discuss pediatric-specific factors related to imaging.

H. Yan
Division of Neurosurgery, University of Toronto, Toronto, ON, Canada
e-mail: han.yan@sickkkids.ca

E. Widjaja
Division of Diagnostic Imaging, Hospital for Sick Children, Toronto, ON, Canada
e-mail: Elysa.Widjaja@sickkids.ca

C. Gorodetsky
Division of Neurology, Hospital for Sick Children, Toronto, ON, Canada
e-mail: Carolina.gorodetsky@sickkids.ca

G. M. Ibrahim (✉)
Division of Neurosurgery, Hospital for Sick Children, Toronto, ON, Canada
e-mail: George.ibrahim@sickkids.ca

A. Boutet, A. M. Lozano (eds.), *Magnetic Resonance Imaging in Deep Brain Stimulation*, https://doi.org/10.1007/978-3-031-16348-7_8

Indications for Pediatric DBS

DBS is most commonly utilized in the treatment of medically refractory movement disorders in pediatric populations such as dystonia and chorea. Increasingly, patients with drug-resistant epilepsy who are not candidates for resective surgery may also consider DBS. The most common indications are listed in Table 8.1.

Dystonia remains one of the most common indications for pediatric DBS. Notably, children with *DYT-TOR1A* related dystonia (DYT1) and other monogenic dystonias (such as *DYT-SGCE*, *DYT-KMT2B* and *GNAO1* related dystonia) respond well to GPi-DBS [3]. Children with neurodegenerative disorders such as pantothenate kinase-associated neurodegeneration (PKAN) and Lesch–Nyhan syndrome (LNS) experience clinically significant improvement post DBS, although the response can be very variable [4, 5]. Individuals with dyskinetic cerebral palsy (CP) have an inferior response to DBS with only 27% having a clinically significant improvement [6]. GPI-DBS should be considered early in the course of refractory status dystonicus as up to 90% of cases resolve after the surgery. In the largest review of pediatric and adolescent patients with dystonia treated with DBS, data from 72 articles and 321 patients demonstrated that 86% of patients showed some improvement with a median motor improvement of 42% [7].

There is increasing impetus to treat patients with dystonia with DBS at younger ages due to the known natural history of the condition, which does not remit over time. Furthermore, recent studies showed that duration of dystonia (shorter time between dystonia diagnosis and DBS surgery) is a significant outcome predictor [8, 9]. Conversely, other movement disorders such as Gilles de la Tourette syndrome (TS) may spontaneously remit without surgery and therefore, DBS ought to be approached with caution for such indications in children [10, 11]. For a subset of children with TS who are adversely affected by the disease, DBS may facilitate social, educational, and brain maturation during critical periods of childhood and adolescence. In a review of 21 articles and 58 pediatric patients with TS, DBS seemed to improve tic severity with 68% of patients demonstrating improvement greater than 50% [12]. Targets of DBS for TS in children were mainly the GPi (57%), although several thalamic targets including the centromedian-parafascicular (CM-Pfc) nuclei have also been attempted.

Children with drug-resistant epilepsy may also be considered DBS candidates. From a review of 21 studies and 40 pediatric patients [13], many DBS targets have

Table 8.1 Summary of common indications and targets of DBS in children

Indication	Targets	Notes
Dystonia/chorea	GPi	High efficiency in monogenic dystonias
Epilepsy	CM-Pfc, ANT	Several common targets with unknown optimal selection. At our institution, we utilize CM for generalized epilepsy specifically Lennox–Gastaut Syndrome (LGS) and ANT for frontal-temporal epilepsy
Tourette syndrome	CM-Pfc, GPi	Controversial due to possibility of disease remission over time

been attempted in children for epilepsy, including the CM-Pfc, the anterior nucleus of the thalamus (ANT), the hippocampus, the subthalamic nucleus (STN), the posteromedial hypothalamus, and the mammillothalamic tract. Although only 12.5% of patients achieved seizure freedom, 85% of the patients were reported to have some seizure frequency reduction.

The indications for pediatric and adolescent DBS will continue to grow as many studies start to assess the perceptions of DBS for children with psychiatric or developmental illness, such as obsessive-compulsive disorder, Rett syndrome, or autism spectrum disorder [(14–16)]. The imaging needs will consequentially also grow as scientists and clinicians try to understand the clinical and radiographic effects of DBS on different populations of children and adolescents.

Imaging Considerations for Children

Although MRI is integral for the planning of all DBS procedures, this is particularly critical for children and adolescents. Indirect targets relative to the anterior commissure-posterior commissure (AC-PC) for localization are based on adult data and therefore may be less accurate in children. Furthermore, it is much more common to perform DBS surgery in children under general anesthesia relative to adults. This may reduce the reliability of microelectrode recordings (MERs) and MRI-based direct targeting becomes crucial for accurate electrode placement. Direct targeting with MRI for children and adolescents also poses additional challenges due to the lack of age-specific atlases. At our institution, postoperative MRI is routinely performed immediately after surgery if general anesthetic is required to acquire a high quality scan. In the subsequent sections, we provide an in-depth review of the many unique aspects of MRI for children and adolescents with DBS.

MR Imaging Acquisition for Planning DBS

The acquisition of high resolution (and therefore time consuming) MRI sequences can prove to be a challenge for some children and adolescents. Certain children are old enough to be aware of the surrounding environment and react to MRI noises but are not cognitively mature to follow instructions, ultimately requiring sedation to acquire adequate scans [17]. Specific diagnostic sequences, such as the spin echo based T2 or echoplanar (EPI) based diffusion, can be difficult to acquire due to relative acquisition time, loud noises, or susceptibility to motion artifacts [18]. We do not propose a specific age cut-off for sedation, but rather individualize this decision to the specific child.

Practically, there are many methods that contribute to the successful acquisition of pediatric MRI scans [18]. First, a dedicated child life team can help to reduce anxiety or claustrophobia for children. These specialists are especially helpful for young or developmentally delayed patients [19, 20]. Second, a practice session with a mock scanner can relax children who are capable of understanding the procedure and rationale of the imaging process [21]. Other options for "MRI practice" include online information for parents, use of toys or stories to simulate the scanning procedure, and virtual reality programs. Third, scans can be broken into manageable 20-to-30-minute segments to allow for breaks when necessary. Last, pediatric-sized MRI scanners can improve image quality by increasing gradient slew rates and decreasing distortion at air tissue interfaces [22]. The ongoing challenges of pediatric neuroimaging are to increase signal to noise while maintaining or shortening scan time.

The acquisition of functional MRI (fMRI) poses additional challenges in children, if these scans are required in research settings before and after DBS. Teamwork and communication between the child life specialist, neuropsychologist, radiologist, and referring physician is critical. In addition, patient comfort and positioning are even more important to optimize given the need to wear headphones and goggles. Pre-fMRI training is often needed to minimize movement and assess for strategies to maintain attention. Yuan et al. [23] found that head movement was greater in younger children and boys when studying various language tasks for fMRI. They report that the use of a visual component or multi-sensory stimulation (i.e., auditory and visual simultaneously) would limit excessive head movement. Pediatric jaws are closer to the brain and would augment movement if tasks require verbal responses, so paradigms should be adjusted accordingly. Reliable and useful fMRI data can be obtained in 95% of typically developing children age 8 and older and 80% of those 4–5 years of age [24]. Unfortunately, patients with cognitive impairment or neuropsychiatric disorders will have a lower rate of fMRI success. In these situations, considerations for resting-state fMRI can still be valuable in assessing intrinsic brain circuitry, as required by the specific study protocols. Real-time fMRI processing is generally recommended to assess for quality during the examination and to allow for repeated attempts. Children have thinner and less muscular skulls, along with shorter necks, which do not always fit readily into MR head coils designed for adults. When the brain does not rest in the center of the head coil, the signal may be distorted by field inhomogeneity reducing the signal to noise ratio upon which activation maps are based [25]. Surface coils closer to the brain are more likely to enhance detection of increased signal induced by blood oxygen level-dependent (BOLD) response [25].

The instigation of these techniques has greatly improved the ability to successfully collect high quality MRI acquisitions in pediatric patients at our institution.

Neuroimaging and the Developing Brain

Between the ages of 2 to early adolescence, total brain matter increases in volume by approximately 25% [26, 27]. The ratio of gray matter and white matter volumes fluctuate as gray matter volumes start decreasing at a younger age compared to white matter volume [28, 29]. Critically, children's brains have more variability than those of adults in shape and size of nuclei [30]. Recognizing these differences is important in the interpretation and analysis of clinical or research data of children or adolescents.

Analyses of pediatric neuroimaging may rely on adult or age-specific atlases or templates. Early data demonstrated that 5-mm resolution of MRI and fMRI images have the ability to transform healthy pediatric brains of age 7–8 within the same stereotactic space as adults' brains [31]. However, the many structural, volumetric, and morphologic differences between adult and pediatric brains have encouraged the development of several pediatric atlases and templates. The Montreal Neurologic Institute (MNI) presented a standard MRI template of brain volume from pediatric data from 324 children age 4.5–18.5 [32]. This was the cumulation of a multi-institutional effort with support from the National Institutes of Health, National Institute of Neurologic Disorders and Stroke, and several other funding agencies. Despite this achievement, there are still many ongoing efforts to develop pediatric templates on larger samples, for specific age ranges, and with updated alignment tools to minimize deformation and optimize resolution [33, 34]. The choice of brain template can have significant impact for structural co-registration when guiding DBS placement (if an atlas is used) and adds to the nuances of pediatric imaging in clinical and research settings.

Several studies have reported that functional activation maps are fundamentally the same in healthy children over the age of 8 and adults [35–38] although greater accuracy can be achieved with age-controlled comparisons. It is possible that during fMRI analysis, one may be overly conservative in the choice of the statistical threshold for pediatric images. Children have a greater gray to white matter ratio, which may increase the threshold relative to adults, although the decreased signal to noise in children may obstruct the real activity from reaching the level of statistical significance [39]. Balancing these considerations requires a team of analysts with experience in pediatric functional imaging.

Clinical Decision-Making for Children Based on Neuroimaging

In the assessment of children with refractory dystonia or epilepsy, a careful review of the child's neuroimaging may yield insights into the etiology of the condition and may allow the clinician to glean some perspectives on whether or not DBS may be successful.

Children with dyskinetic forms of cerebral palsy (CP) may demonstrate abnormal findings within the deep gray structures due to injury from hypoxic insult [40]. Extensive injury to the GPi may yield GPi-DBS less effective, although at present, there are no clear criteria to the extent of injury that would preclude a child from undergoing the procedure. Ongoing studies evaluating preoperative neuroimaging biomarkers of treatment success will likely inform such decision-making in the future [35].

Functional neuroimaging may also better define the subtypes of CP, given that many children present with "mixed patterns" (most frequently co-existence of dystonia and spasticity) [41]. Specifically, diffusion tensor imaging (DTI) provides details regarding white matter microstructure. White matter injury is the most common imaging finding for all children with CP, and commonly seen in children with spastic CP subtypes. This could inform preoperative patient stratification. For instance, Lumsden et al. [42] suggest that differences in the fractional anisotropy (FA) between children inherited and acquired dystonia could account for different responses to DBS. In surgical decision-making for DBS candidates with dystonia, neuroimaging remains a critical factor to determine eligibility for surgery and perhaps also predict effectiveness of treatment.

Although there are established guidelines for the diagnosis and treatment of pediatric epilepsy [43], there is significant heterogeneity in the image acquisition protocols. The HARNESS-MRI protocol of 2019 [44] proposes the following mandatory sequences: magnetization-prepared rapid gradient-echo (MPRAGE), 3D fluid attenuation inversion recovery (FLAIR), and coronal spin echo with the long axis perpendicular to the hippocampus. Optional sequences include gadolinium-enhanced MRI and susceptibility weighted imaging. These sequences are necessary to evaluate for hippocampal sclerosis, brain tumors, and malformations of cortical development, vascular malformations, glial scars or encephalitis that may help determine if a resective surgical approach would be appropriate.

Children and adolescents with epilepsy presenting for consideration of DBS may have no apparent lesion on MRI. This is not surprising, given that approximately 50% of children with epilepsy present with no visible pathology on MRI [45, 46]. It is unknown if normal thalamic or thalamocortical anatomy is a requirement for DBS eligibility, and there are no clear exclusion criteria to delineate the relative degree of thalamic injury that would preclude CM or ANT surgery. Both fMRI and DTI will likely prove to be critical in the understanding of epileptic networks and seizure propagation and the effect of neuromodulation on brain network excitability.

DBS Targeting in Children

DBS for children differs in technique from the adult surgery for several reasons, including the fact that children are often placed under general anesthetic for electrode implantation. Although it is possible to record robust MERs under general anesthetic, it may limit their utility. Furthermore, in children with dystonia and epilepsy, there are no immediate on-off effects that can be tested intraoperatively. Adverse stimulation effects on the cortical spinal tract in the form of unintended contractures are often assessed when inserting electrodes in GPi, which provides some insights into the medial and posterior boundaries of the electrode positions. In children undergoing CM-DBS, we routinely attempt to capture a recruiting rhythm in response to stimulation using intraoperative scalp electroencephalography. It has been shown that low frequency stimulation of the CM generates a recruiting rhythm causing EEG synchronization and high frequency stimulation leads to desynchronization [47, 48]. Stimulation of the CM-Pfc has also been described to desynchronize intractable focal seizures with motor onset in adult stereoelectroencephalographic patients [49]. Alongside direct MR targeting, these techniques in children are helpful for confirmation of accurate electrode placement.

Certain sequences have been optimized at the Hospital for Sick Children in Toronto to help with direct targeting in the planning stages of DBS implantation (Table 8.2). Although the resolution and contrast can be adjusted to help delineate the target nuclei, the exact borders often remain challenging to define. Knowledge of neighboring structures and the relative intensities of nuclei are important for assessment of a direct target.

Direct and indirect targeting methods are both utilized to optimize the placement of DBS electrodes in children. In children, indirect formulaic targeting is not appropriate as a singular approach and direct targeting of visualized structures is preferred. In children with dystonia, Vayssiere et al. [50] have demonstrated that MRI distortions did not induce detectable errors during stereotactic surgery and that MRI-based target localization alone produced acceptable clinical results. In a recent study of DBS for children with dystonia [51], the authors utilized direct GPi targeting in addition to MERs to elucidate substrates underlying clinical outcome. Volume of tissue activated (VTA)-based probabilistic mapping suggested DBS-induced benefits within the posterior GPi, lateral and significantly superior to the widely described target in adults by Horn et al. [52] The authors report the optimized 50% of voxels were centered on the following MNI coordinates: $x = 23.7$, $y = -9.4$, $z = -3.7$ [51]. This area has 59.3% overlap with the GPi proper, greatest in the premotor and primary motor territories, with 29.8% overlap with the globus pallidus pars externa (GPe). While preliminary, pediatric-focused neuroimaging studies of DBS patients may demonstrate slight variances between optimal hot-spots for DBS in the developing brain when compared to adults.

Table 8.2 Optimized parameters of MRI sequences to aid in direct targeting for DBS

Sequence	Parameters on Philips 3 T Achieva	Parameters on Siemens 3 T Skyra
Axial 3D T1	TR/TE = 6.0/2.7 msec, FOV = 22 cm, TSE = 213, Flip angle = 8°, voxel size = 0.45 × 0.45 × 0.45 mm	TR/TE = 1640/2.38 msec, FOV = 22 cm, TI = 800 msec, Flip angle = 8°, voxel size = 0.45 × 0.45 × 0.5 mm
Axial T2	TR/TE = 3000/287 msec, FOV = 22 cm, TSE = 145, Flip angle 60°, voxel size = 0.7 × 0.7 × 1.0 mm, SENSE = 1.7	TR/TE = 4070/81 msec, FOV = 22 cm, Flip angle = 150°, matrix = 213 × 320, slice thickness = 1.2 mm, IPAT = 2
Axial STIR	TR/TE = 10,363/210 msec, FOV = 22 cm, TSE = 17, Flip angle = 120°, matrix = 316x278, slice thickness = 1 mm, SENSE = 1.8	TR/TE = 7850/72 msec, FOV = 22 cm, TI = 150 msec, Flip angle = 140°, matrix = 256x256, slice thickness = 1 mm, IPAT = 2
Sagittal 3D FLAIR	TR/TE = 8000/335 msec, FOV = 22 cm, TSE = 110, IR = 2400 msec, Flip angle = 50°, voxel = 1.2 × 1.2 × 1.2 mm, SENSE = 2	TR/TE = 5000/387 msec, FOV = 23 cm, TI = 1600 msec, voxel = 0.4 × 0.4 × 0.9 mm, IPAT = 2

Postoperative DBS Imaging

The postoperative DBS images are important to establish correct placement and may aid in the subsequent programming of the electrodes. The sequences for post-operative DBS at the Hospital for Sick Children are provided in Table 8.3. We do not recommend serial imaging for young children with DBS. Electrode migration due to growth of a developing brain can be suspected if there is an unexpected change in the response of DBS after years of stability on specific stimulation parameters. A comparison of preoperative and postoperative images of GPi and CM-Pfc are shown in Figs. 8.1 and 8.2, respectively.

Table 8.3 Parameters of MRI sequences for postoperative DBS

Sequence	Parameters on Siemens 3 T Skyra
Axial 3D T1	TR/TE = 1830/3.78 msec, FOV = 22 cm, TI = 800 msec, Flip angle = 8°, voxel size = 1.0 × 1.0 × 1.0 mm
Axial T2	TR/TE = 4470/96 msec, FOV = 22 cm, Flip angle = 90°, matrix = 186x256, slice thickness = 3 mm, NEX = 2
Coronal T2	TR/TE = 5300/108 msec, FOV = 22 cm, Flip angle = 90°, matrix = 186 × 256, slice thickness = 3 mm, NEX = 2

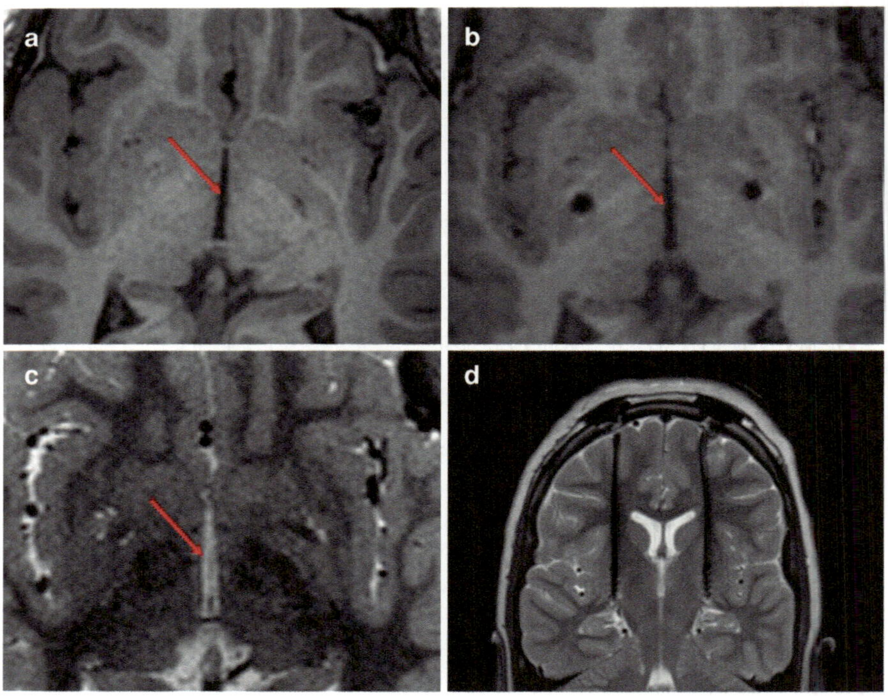

Fig. 8.1 Preoperative and postoperative images of GPi-DBS. (**a**) Preoperative T1-weighted image. (**b**) Preoperative STIR image with adjusted resolution of nuclei. (**c**) T2-weighted postoperative axial image showing placement of the GPi electrode tips. (**d**) T2-weighted adjusted coronal image along the electrode trajectory. The red arrow shows the mid-commissural point. *DBS* deep brain stimulation, *GPi* globus pallidus internus, *STIR* short tau inversion recovery

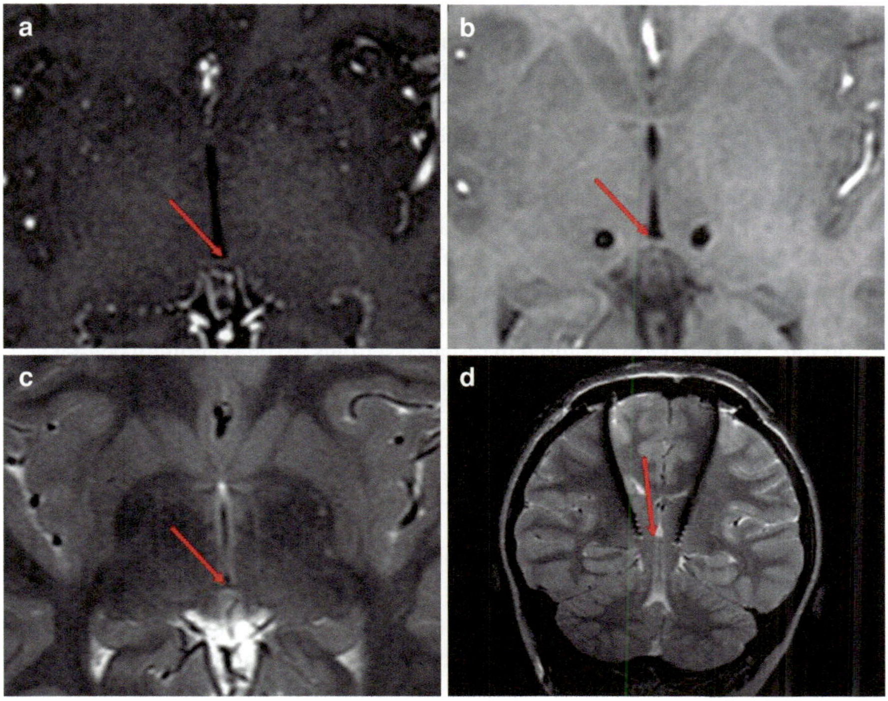

Fig. 8.2 Preoperative and postoperative images of CM-Pfc DBS. (**a**) T1-weighted preoperative image. (**b**) T2-weighted preoperative image with improved resolution of nuclei. (**c**) T2-weighted postoperative axial image showing placement of the CM-Pfc electrode tips. (**d**) T2-weighted adjusted coronal image along the electrode trajectory. The red arrow shows the posterior commissure. CM-Pfc = centromedian-parafascicular

Ethics of Pediatric DBS and Neuroimaging

Relative to DBS for adults, pediatric DBS is still an emerging field for clinicians and researchers, concentrated only at a handful of centers. Involvement of children in decisions to undergo DBS treatment or to enter into a neuroimaging study can be difficult since not all children are able to declare their preferences due to immaturity or lack of cognitive abilities. Furthermore, the stress of any procedure, be it MRI or surgery, cannot be reliably predicted in children. It is critical to prioritize the child's best interest in all decisions surrounding DBS, including the acquisition of neuroimaging. A set of guidelines have been published with regard to the ethical conduct of DBS in children [53]. These guidelines advocate for (i) care in the design and conduct of clinical research studies, emphasizing the child's best interest, (ii) the prioritization of the child's developmental context when approaching hypotheses and outcomes, (iii) cautious application of adult data to the design of pediatric trials, and (iv) diligent reporting of methods and results in the spirit of collaboration. These same guidelines should be applied in the conduct of neuroimaging in a clinical and research context surrounding pediatric DBS. Neuroimaging correlated with clinical outcomes across several institutions will be critical to understand anatomy and networks that either contribute to effective treatment or trigger unwanted side effects. A multi-institutional prospective, comprehensive registry for pediatric DBS, the CHILD-DBS database is actively collecting both clinical and neuroimaging data with a view towards better understanding the effects of DBS on pathologies affecting the developing brain [54].

Finally, although the harms of MRI acquisition in children are generally low, several bioethical questions were posed for participants of observational neuroimaging studies of children and adolescents [55]. These include issues surrounding the disclosure of incidental findings and clinical reporting of sensitive information involving risky behaviors acquired in research settings. Even seemingly benign neuroimaging research studies can be complicated by bioethical questions that require careful consideration and foresight.

Conclusions

Although DBS may still be considered a relatively novel treatment option for children, this procedure is supported by decades of clinical experience and data from adult populations. The conduct of DBS in children and adolescents is associated with unique considerations that call for the cautious adaptation of adult protocols and evidence. As the number of indications for DBS in pediatric populations grows, so do neuroimaging need for both clinical and research purposes.

On the basis of our experience in pediatric DBS, the current chapter provided several considerations related to neuroimaging in children and adolescents, from MRI acquisition to analysis and interpretation. It is evident that greater knowledge linking the effects of DBS to pathologies that affect the developing brain will inform clinical decision-making for the conduct of these procedures in pediatric populations. Advanced neuroimaging techniques including fMRI and DTI will continue to play a meaningful role in better understanding these associations. Multi-institutional collaboration among centers performing pediatric DBS will be critical to combine expertise and improve the care provided to children and adolescents.

References

1. Coubes P, Echenne B, Roubertie A, Vayssiere N, Tuffery S, Humbertclaude V, et al. Treatment of early-onset generalized dystonia by chronic bilateral stimulation of the internal globus pallidus. Apropos of a case. Neurochirurgie. 1999;45(2):139–44.
2. Cif L, Coubes P. Historical developments in children's deep brain stimulation. Eur J Paediatr Neurol. 2017;21(1):109–17.
3. Phukan J, Albanese A, Gasser T, Warner T. Primary dystonia and dystonia-plus syndromes: clinical characteristics, diagnosis, and pathogenesis. Lancet Neurol. 2011;10(12):1074–85.
4. Tambirajoo K, Furlanetti L, Hasegawa H, Raslan A, Gimeno H, Lin JP, et al. Deep brain stimulation of the internal pallidum in Lesch-Nyhan syndrome: clinical outcomes and connectivity analysis. Neuromodulation. 2021;24(2):380–91.

5. Svetel M, Tomic A, Dragasevic N, Petrovic I, Kresojevic N, Jech R, et al. Clinical course of patients with pantothenate kinase-associated neurodegeneration (PKAN) before and after DBS surgery. J Neurol. 2019;266(12):2962–9.
6. Bohn E, Goren K, Switzer L, Falck-Ytter Y, Fehlings D. Pharmacological and neurosurgical interventions for individuals with cerebral palsy and dystonia: a systematic review update and meta-analysis. Dev Med Child Neurol. 2021;63(9):1038–50.
7. Elkaim LM, Alotaibi NM, Sigal A, Alotaibi HM, Lipsman N, Kalia SK, et al. Deep brain stimulation for pediatric dystonia: a meta-analysis with individual participant data. Dev Med Child Neurol. 2019;61(1):49–56.
8. Lumsden DE, Kaminska M, Gimeno H, Tustin K, Baker L, Perides S, et al. Proportion of life lived with dystonia inversely correlates with response to pallidal deep brain stimulation in both primary and secondary childhood dystonia. Dev Med Child Neurol. 2013;55(6): 567–74.
9. Vasques X, Cif L, Gonzalez V, Nicholson C, Coubes P. Factors predicting improvement in primary generalized dystonia treated by pallidal deep brain stimulation. Mov Disord. 2009;24(6):846–53.
10. Mink JW, Walkup J, Frey KA, Como P, Cath D, Delong MR, et al. Patient selection and assessment recommendations for deep brain stimulation in Tourette syndrome. Mov Disord. 2006;21(11):1831–8.
11. Smeets A, Duits AA, Horstkotter D, Verdellen C, de Wert G, Temel Y, et al. Ethics of deep brain stimulation in adolescent patients with refractory Tourette syndrome: a systematic review and two case discussions. Neuroethics. 2018;11(2):143–55.
12. Coulombe MA, Elkaim LM, Alotaibi NM, Gorman DA, Weil AG, Fallah A, et al. Deep brain stimulation for Gilles de la Tourette syndrome in children and youth: a meta-analysis with individual participant data. J Neurosurg Pediatr. 2018;23(2):236–46.
13. Yan H, Toyota E, Anderson M, Abel TJ, Donner E, Kalia SK, et al. A systematic review of deep brain stimulation for the treatment of drug-resistant epilepsy in childhood. J Neurosurg Pediatr. 2018;23(3):274–84.
14. Munoz KA, Kostick K, Torgerson L, Zuk P, Kalwani L, Sanchez C, et al. Pressing ethical issues in considering pediatric deep brain stimulation for obsessive-compulsive disorder. Brain Stimul. 2021;14(6):1566–72.
15. Storch EA, Cepeda SL, Lee E, Goodman SLV, Robinson AD, De Nadai AS, et al. Parental attitudes toward deep brain stimulation in adolescents with treatment-resistant conditions. J Child Adolesc Psychopharmacol. 2020;30(2):97–103.
16. Weinzimmer SA, Schneider SC, Cepeda SL, Guzick AG, Lazaro-Munoz G, McIngvale E, et al. Perceptions of deep brain stimulation for adolescents with obsessive-compulsive disorder. J Child Adolesc Psychopharmacol. 2021;31(2):109–17.
17. Barkovich MJ, Li Y, Desikan RS, Barkovich AJ, Xu D. Challenges in pediatric neuroimaging. NeuroImage. 2019;185:793–801.
18. Barkovich MJ, Xu D, Desikan RS, Williams C, Barkovich AJ. Pediatric neuro MRI: tricks to minimize sedation. Pediatr Radiol. 2018;48(1):50–5.
19. Durand DJ, Young M, Nagy P, Tekes A, Huisman TA. Mandatory child life consultation and its impact on pediatric MRI workflow in an Academic Medical Center. J Am Coll Radiol. 2015;12(6):594–8.
20. Thieba C, Frayne A, Walton M, Mah A, Benischek A, Dewey D, et al. Factors associated with successful MRI scanning in unsedated young children. Front Pediatr. 2018;6:146.
21. de Bie HM, Boersma M, Wattjes MP, Adriaanse S, Vermeulen RJ, Oostrom KJ, et al. Preparing children with a mock scanner training protocol results in high quality structural and functional MRI scans. Eur J Pediatr. 2010;169(9):1079–85.
22. Weavers PT, Shu Y, Tao S, Huston J 3rd, Lee SK, Graziani D, et al. Technical note: compact three-tesla magnetic resonance imager with high-performance gradients passes ACR image quality and acoustic noise tests. Med Phys. 2016;43(3):1259–64.
23. Yuan W, Altaye M, Ret J, Schmithorst V, Byars AW, Plante E, et al. Quantification of head motion in children during various fMRI language tasks. Hum Brain Mapp 2009;30(5):1481–9.

24. O'Shaughnessy ES, Berl MM, Moore EN, Gaillard WD. Pediatric functional magnetic resonance imaging (fMRI): issues and applications. J Child Neurol. 2008;23(7):791–801.
25. Gaillard WD, Hertz-Pannier L, Mott SH, Barnett AS, LeBihan D, Theodore WH. Functional anatomy of cognitive development: fMRI of verbal fluency in children and adults. Neurology. 2000;54(1):180–5.
26. Caviness VS Jr, Kennedy DN, Richelme C, Rademacher J, Filipek PA. The human brain age 7-11 years: a volumetric analysis based on magnetic resonance images. Cereb Cortex. 1996;6(5):726–36.
27. Miguel PM, Pereira LO, Silveira PP, Meaney MJ. Early environmental influences on the development of children's brain structure and function. Dev Med Child Neurol. 2019;61(10):1127–33.
28. Benedetti B, Charil A, Rovaris M, Judica E, Valsasina P, Sormani MP, et al. Influence of aging on brain gray and white matter changes assessed by conventional, MT, and DT MRI. Neurology. 2006;66(4):535–9.
29. Pfefferbaum A, Mathalon DH, Sullivan EV, Rawles JM, Zipursky RB, Lim KO. A quantitative magnetic resonance imaging study of changes in brain morphology from infancy to late adulthood. Arch Neurol. 1994;51(9):874–87.
30. Oschwald J, Guye S, Liem F, Rast P, Willis S, Rocke C, et al. Brain structure and cognitive ability in healthy aging: a review on longitudinal correlated change. Rev Neurosci. 2019;31(1):1–57.
31. Burgund ED, Kang HC, Kelly JE, Buckner RL, Snyder AZ, Petersen SE, et al. The feasibility of a common stereotactic space for children and adults in fMRI studies of development. NeuroImage. 2002;17(1):184–200.
32. Fonov V, Evans AC, Botteron K, Almli CR, McKinstry RC, Collins DL, et al. Unbiased average age-appropriate atlases for pediatric studies. NeuroImage. 2011;54(1):313–27.
33. Huang CM, Lee SH, Hsiao IT, Kuan WC, Wai YY, Ko HJ, et al. Study-specific EPI template improves group analysis in functional MRI of young and older adults. J Neurosci Methods. 2010;189(2):257–66.
34. Molfese PJ, Glen D, Mesite L, Cox RW, Hoeft F, Frost SJ, et al. The Haskins pediatric atlas: a magnetic-resonance-imaging-based pediatric template and atlas. Pediatr Radiol. 2021;51(4):628–39.
35. Aravamuthan BR, Waugh JL. Localization of basal ganglia and thalamic damage in dyskinetic cerebral palsy. Pediatr Neurol. 2016;54:11–21.
36. Lee BC, Kuppusamy K, Grueneich R, El-Ghazzawy O, Gordon RE, Lin W, et al. Hemispheric language dominance in children demonstrated by functional magnetic resonance imaging. J Child Neurol. 1999;14(2):78–82.
37. Meinhold T, Hofer W, Pieper T, Kudernatsch M, Staudt M. Presurgical language fMRI in children, adolescents and Young adults : a validation study. Clin Neuroradiol. 2020;30(4):691–704.
38. Thomas KM, King SW, Franzen PL, Welsh TF, Berkowitz AL, Noll DC, et al. A developmental functional MRI study of spatial working memory. NeuroImage. 1999;10(3 Pt 1):327–38.
39. Gaillard WD, Grandin CB, Xu B. Developmental aspects of pediatric fMRI: considerations for image acquisition, analysis, and interpretation. NeuroImage. 2001;13(2):239–49.
40. Martinez-Biarge M, Diez-Sebastian J, Kapellou O, Gindner D, Allsop JM, Rutherford MA, et al. Predicting motor outcome and death in term hypoxic-ischemic encephalopathy. Neurology. 2011;76(24):2055–61.
41. Reid SM, Carlin JB, Reddihough DS. Distribution of motor types in cerebral palsy: how do registry data compare? Dev Med Child Neurol. 2011;53(3):233–8.
42. Lumsden DE, Ashmore J, Ball G, Charles-Edwards G, Selway R, Ashkan K, et al. Fractional anisotropy in children with dystonia or spasticity correlates with the selection for DBS or ITB movement disorder surgery. Neuroradiology. 2016;58(4):401–8.
43. Reid SM, Dagia CD, Ditchfield MR, Carlin JB, Reddihough DS. Population-based studies of brain imaging patterns in cerebral palsy. Dev Med Child Neurol. 2014;56(3):222–32.
44. Bernasconi A, Cendes F, Theodore WH, Gill RS, Koepp MJ, Hogan RE, et al. Recommendations for the use of structural magnetic resonance imaging in the care of patients with epilepsy:

a consensus report from the international league against epilepsy neuroimaging task force. Epilepsia. 2019;60(6):1054–68.
45. Bernasconi A, Bernasconi N, Bernhardt BC, Schrader D. Advances in MRI for 'cryptogenic' epilepsies. Nat Rev Neurol. 2011;7(2):99–108.
46. Wang I, Bernasconi A, Bernhardt B, Blumenfeld H, Cendes F, Chinvarun Y, et al. MRI essentials in epileptology: a review from the ILAE imaging taskforce. Epileptic Disord. 2020;22(4):421–37.
47. Cukiert A, Lehtimaki K. Deep brain stimulation targeting in refractory epilepsy. Epilepsia. 2017;58(Suppl 1):80–4.
48. Jaseja H, Gupta A, Jain R, Gupta P. Intractable epilepsy: deep brain stimulation (DBS)-based electrophysiological biomarker. Epilepsy Behav. 2014;31:13–4.
49. Chkhenkeli SA, Sramka M, Lortkipanidze GS, Rakviashvili TN, Bregvadze E, Magalashvili GE, et al. Electrophysiological effects and clinical results of direct brain stimulation for intractable epilepsy. Clin Neurol Neurosurg. 2004;106(4):318–29.
50. Vayssiere N, Hemm S, Zanca M, Picot MC, Bonafe A, Cif L, et al. Magnetic resonance imaging stereotactic target localization for deep brain stimulation in dystonic children. J Neurosurg. 2000;93(5):784–90.
51. Coblentz A, Elias GJB, Boutet A, Germann J, Algarni M, Oliveira LM, et al. Mapping efficacious deep brain stimulation for pediatric dystonia. J Neurosurg Pediatr. 2021:1–11.
52. Horn A, Kuhn AA, Merkl A, Shih L, Alterman R, Fox M. Probabilistic conversion of neurosurgical DBS electrode coordinates into MNI space. NeuroImage. 2017;150 395–404.
53. Davidson B, Elkaim LM, Lipsman N, Ibrahim GM. Editorial. An ethical framework for deep brain stimulation in children. Neurosurg Focus. 2018;45(3):E11.
54. Yan H, Siegel L, Breitbart S, Gorodetsky C, Gonorazky HD, Yau I, et al. The Child & Youth CompreHensIve longitudinal database for deep brain stimulation (CHILD-DBS). Childs Nerv Syst. 2021;37(2):607–15.
55. Clark DB, Fisher CB, Bookheimer S, Brown SA, Evans JH, Hopfer C, et al. Biomedical ethics and clinical oversight in multisite observational neuroimaging studies with children and adolescents: the ABCD experience. Dev Cogn Neurosci. 2018;32:143–54.

9 Deep Brain Stimulation and Magnetic Resonance Imaging: Future Directions

Alexandre Boutet and Andres M. Lozano

The increasingly available ultra-high-field 7.0 Tesla MRI represents a major advancement [1, 2]. It offers unprecedented image resolution, permitting the delineation of smaller neuroanatomical structures. Once current limitations such as increased image distortion have been addressed, direct targeting with ultra-high-field MRI will likely emerge as the dominant surgical planning technique. Coil and gradient developments will lead to improved and novel pulse sequences further enhancing target visualization. Towards network-based connectomic targeting, we believe advanced sequences visualizing larger networks rather than discrete structures will become increasingly prominent [3]. In contrast to the indirect targeting techniques that have traditionally dominated stereotactic neurosurgery, these novel MRI targeting methods will open the door to individualized surgical planning, allowing symptom-specific *circuitopathies* to be precisely modulated based on patients' most disabling symptoms and thereby maximizing quality of life improvement [4–6].

With regard to imaging patients with fully implanted devices, we expect that the DBS hardware will become more "imaging friendly" with increased MRI compatibility and decreased metallic susceptibility artefact [7]. This is necessary as MRI becomes the gold standard imaging modality for a growing number of indications and as it continues to develop as a pivotal component in many research endeavours. As such, MRI compatibility will become a particularly important element of marketing for vendors. We also anticipate vendors and researchers to start investigating the safety of 7.0 Tesla MRI in DBS patients due to its potential to be

A. Boutet (✉)
Joint Department of Medical Imaging, University of Toronto, Toronto, ON, Canada
e-mail: alexandre.boutet@mail.utoronto.ca

A. M. Lozano
Division of Neurosurgery, University Health Network and University of Toronto, Toronto, ON, Canada
e-mail: lozano@uhnresearch.ca

A. Boutet, A. M. Lozano (eds.), *Magnetic Resonance Imaging in Deep Brain Stimulation*, https://doi.org/10.1007/978-3-031-16348-7_9

used as a powerful research and clinical tool. Individuals receiving DBS will benefit from this additional MRI safety knowledge as it offers the potential to expand the possibilities of MRI and provide further research tools.

We predict that this expanded role of MRI in DBS will lead the way towards imaging-based biomarkers, which will address pressing issues such as patient selection and postoperative programming. Functional MRI (fMRI) has been put forward as a rapid and objective biomarker of treatment success for motor and psychiatric DBS indications [8–10]. Such a tool could facilitate individualized medicine for these patients and may represent a step towards the possibility of autonomous, closed-loop DBS programming. Finally, it is important to continue learning from past DBS interventions with group-level MRI-based probabilistic stimulation mapping techniques, as they allow clinicians to refine current targeting and also lay the groundwork for new network-based connectomics [11, 12].

In summary, we envisage a future in which the role of MRI in DBS will continue to expand. It will likely be part of most future clinical and research endeavours, meaning that familiarity with this tool and a firm understanding of its usages will become an essential skill.

References

1. Boutet A, Gramer R, Steele CJ, Elias GJB, Germann J, Maciel R, et al. Neuroimaging technological advancements for targeting in functional neurosurgery. Curr Neurol Neurosci Rep. 2019;19(7):42.
2. Forstmann BU, Isaacs BR, Temel Y. Ultra high field MRI-guided deep brain stimulation. Trends Biotechnol. 2017;35(10):904–7.
3. Coenen VA, Reisert M. DTI for brain targeting: diffusion weighted imaging fiber tractography-assisted deep brain stimulation. Int Rev Neurobiol. 2021;159:47–67.
4. Baldermann JC, Melzer C, Zapf A, Kohl S, Timmermann L, Tittgemeyer M, et al. Connectivity profile predictive of effective deep brain stimulation in obsessive-compulsive disorder. Biol Psychiatry. 2019;85(9):735–43.
5. Boutet A, Germann J, Gwun D, Loh A, Elias GJB, Neudorfer C, et al. Sign-specific stimulation 'hot' and 'cold' spots in Parkinson's disease validated with machine learning. Brain Commun. 2021;3(2):fcab027.
6. Lozano AM, Lipsman N. Probing and regulating dysfunctional circuits using deep brain stimulation. Neuron. 2013;77(3):406–24.
7. Boutet A, Chow CT, Narang K, Elias GJB, Neudorfer C, Germann J, et al. Improving safety of MRI in patients with deep brain stimulation devices. Radiology. 2020;296(2):250–62.
8. Boutet A, Madhavan R, Elias GJB, Joel SE, Gramer R, Ranjan M, et al. Predicting optimal deep brain stimulation parameters for Parkinson's disease using functional MRI and machine learning. Nat Commun. 2021;12(1):3043.
9. Elias GJB, Germann J, Boutet A, Loh A, Li B, Pancholi A, et al. 3T MRI of rapid brain activity changes driven by subcallosal cingulate deep brain stimulation. Brain. 2022;145(6):2214–26.
10. Loh A, Elias GJB, Germann J, Boutet A, Gwun D, Yamamoto K, et al. Neural correlates of optimal deep brain stimulation for cervical dystonia. Ann Neurol. 2022;92(3):418–24.
11. Horn A, Reich M, Vorwerk J, Li N, Wenzel G, Fang Q, et al. Connectivity predicts deep brain stimulation outcome in Parkinson disease. Ann Neurol. 2017;82(1):67–78.
12. Elias GJB, Boutet A, Joel SE, Germann J, Gwun D, Neudorfer C, et al. Probabilistic mapping of deep brain stimulation: insights from 15 years of therapy. Ann Neurol. 2021;89(3):426–43.

Index

A. Boutet, A. M. Lozano (eds.), *Magnetic Resonance Imaging in Deep Brain Stimulation*, https://doi.org/10.1007/978-3-031-16348-7

GPSR Compliance

The European Union's (EU) General Product Safety Regulation (GPSR) is a set of rules that requires consumer products to be safe and our obligations to ensure this.

If you have any concerns about our products, you can contact us on ProductSafety@springernature.com

In case Publisher is established outside the EU, the EU authorized representative is:

Springer Nature Customer Service Center GmbH
Europaplatz 3
69115 Heidelberg, Germany

Batch number: 10166020

Printed by Printforce, the Netherlands